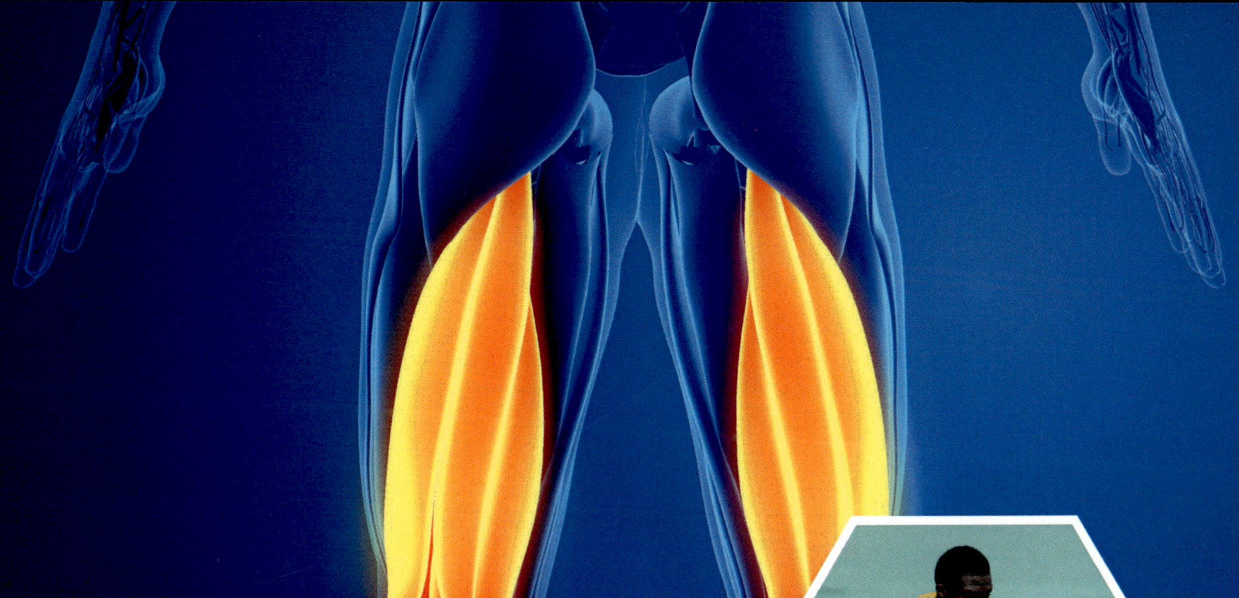

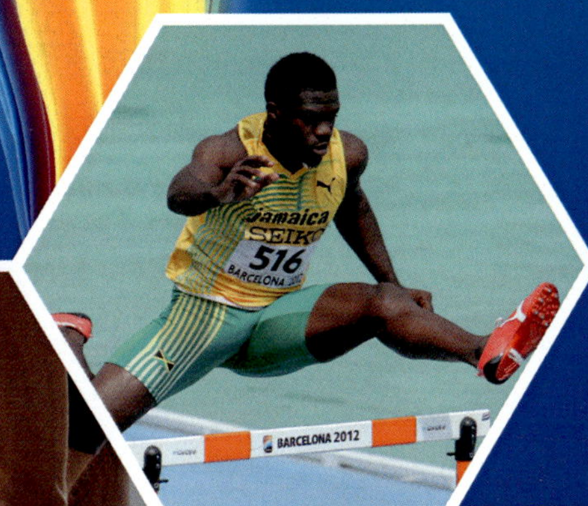

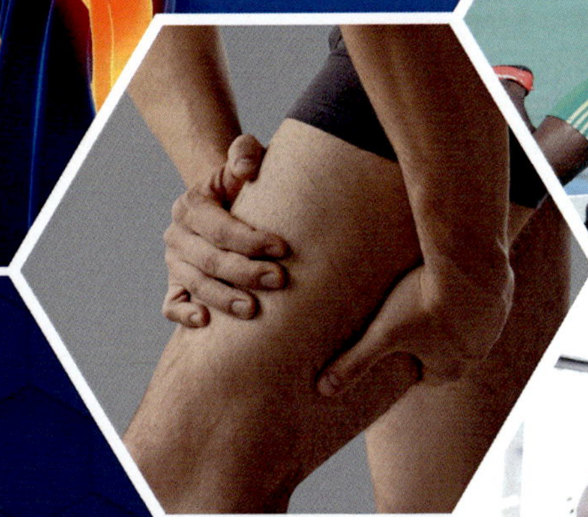

India James

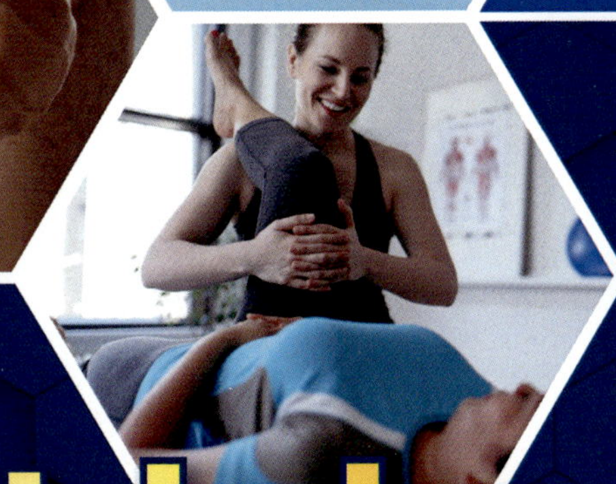

SPORTS INJURIES

Hamstring Injuries

A Crabtree Forest Book

Crabtree Publishing

crabtreebooks.com

School-to-Home Support for Caregivers and Teachers

This appealing book is designed to teach students about core subject areas. Students will build upon what they already know about the subject and engage in topics that they want to learn more about. Here are a few guiding questions to help readers build comprehension skills. Possible answers appear here in red.

Before Reading:

- What do I know about hamstring injuries?
  - *I know that many athletes get hamstring injuries*
  - *I know that hamstring injuries happen in your leg*
- What do I want to learn about this topic?
  - *I want to know what muscles get hamstring injuries*
  - *I want to know how to prevent hamstring injuries*

During Reading:

- I'm curious to know...
  - *I'm curious to know what I may feel like after a hamstring injury*
  - *I'm curious to know what might happen at a doctor's office after a hamstring injury*
- How is this like something I already know?
  - *I know that hamstring injuries often happen while running*
  - *I know that hamstring injuries sometimes happen to athletes more than once*

After Reading:

- What was the author trying to teach me?
  - *The author was trying to teach me what parts of my body are hurt by hamstring injuries*
  - *The author was trying to teach me that there are ways to help prevent hamstring injuries*
- How did the photographs and captions help me understand more?
  - *The drawings of leg muscles and bones helped me to understand the muscles and bones of the hamstring complex*
  - *The pictures of MRI, X-ray, and ultrasound machines helped me understand what tests a doctor might use to understand my hamstring injury.*

Table of Contents

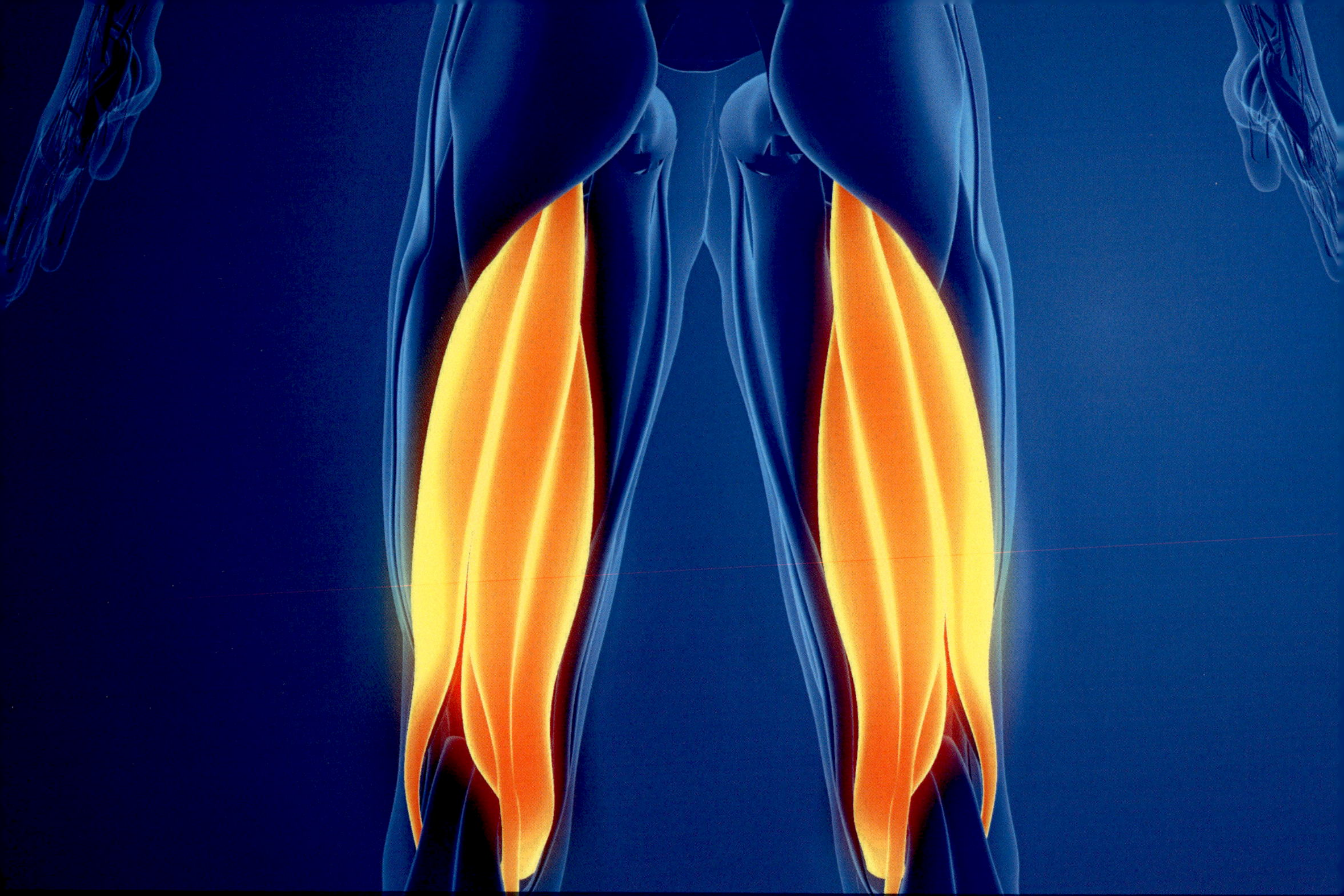

Chapter 1: What Are Hamstring Injuries?

The sprinter speeds down the track. Her hands whip back and forth as her legs take long, powerful strides down the green, rubber surface. Then, all of a sudden, she collapses. She didn't trip, and she didn't hit any other runners. What happened?

The basketball player dribbles down the court. He fakes left and cuts rights, running past the defender. Then, he falls to the ground, clutching at the back of his leg. He didn't stumble, and he wasn't fouled by any other player. What happened?

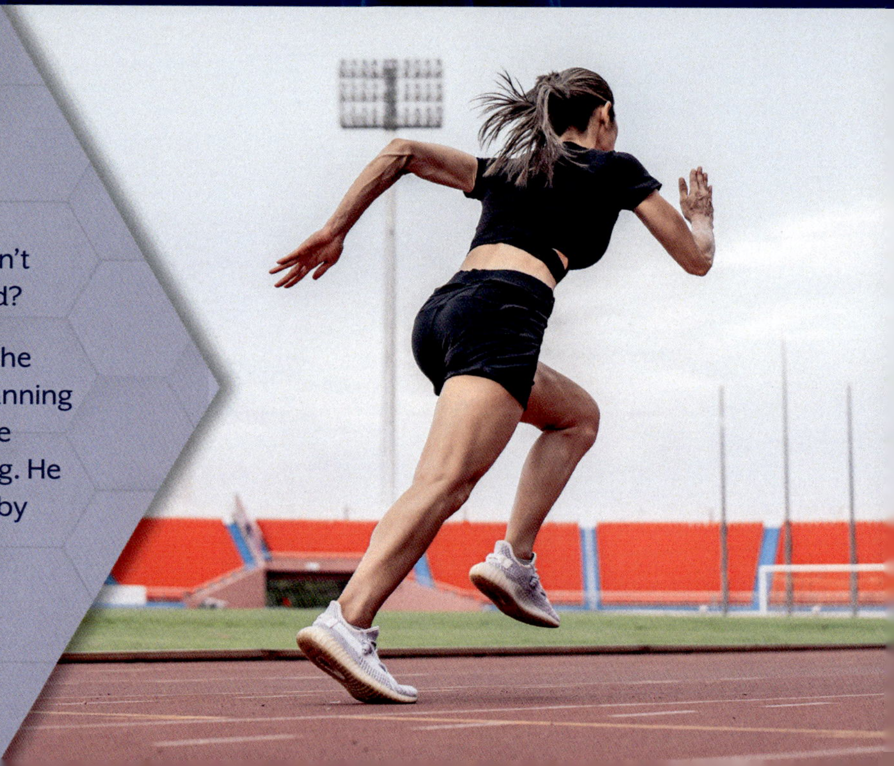

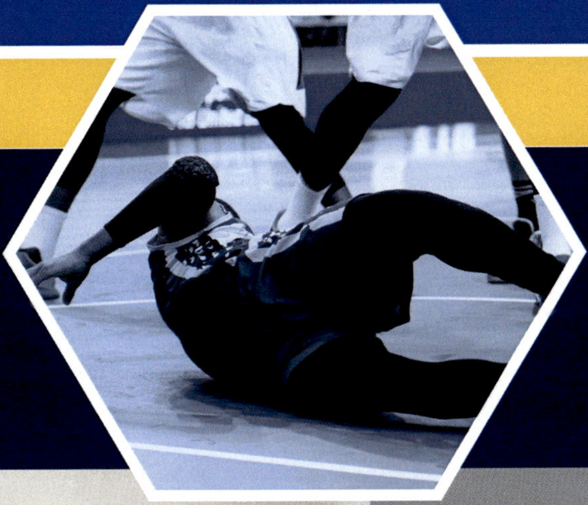

Hamstring Injuries

Both of these athletes hurt their hamstrings. The hamstrings are a group of three muscles in the back of the leg. Injuries to the hamstring muscles happen when one or more of the muscles is pulled too far and becomes strained.

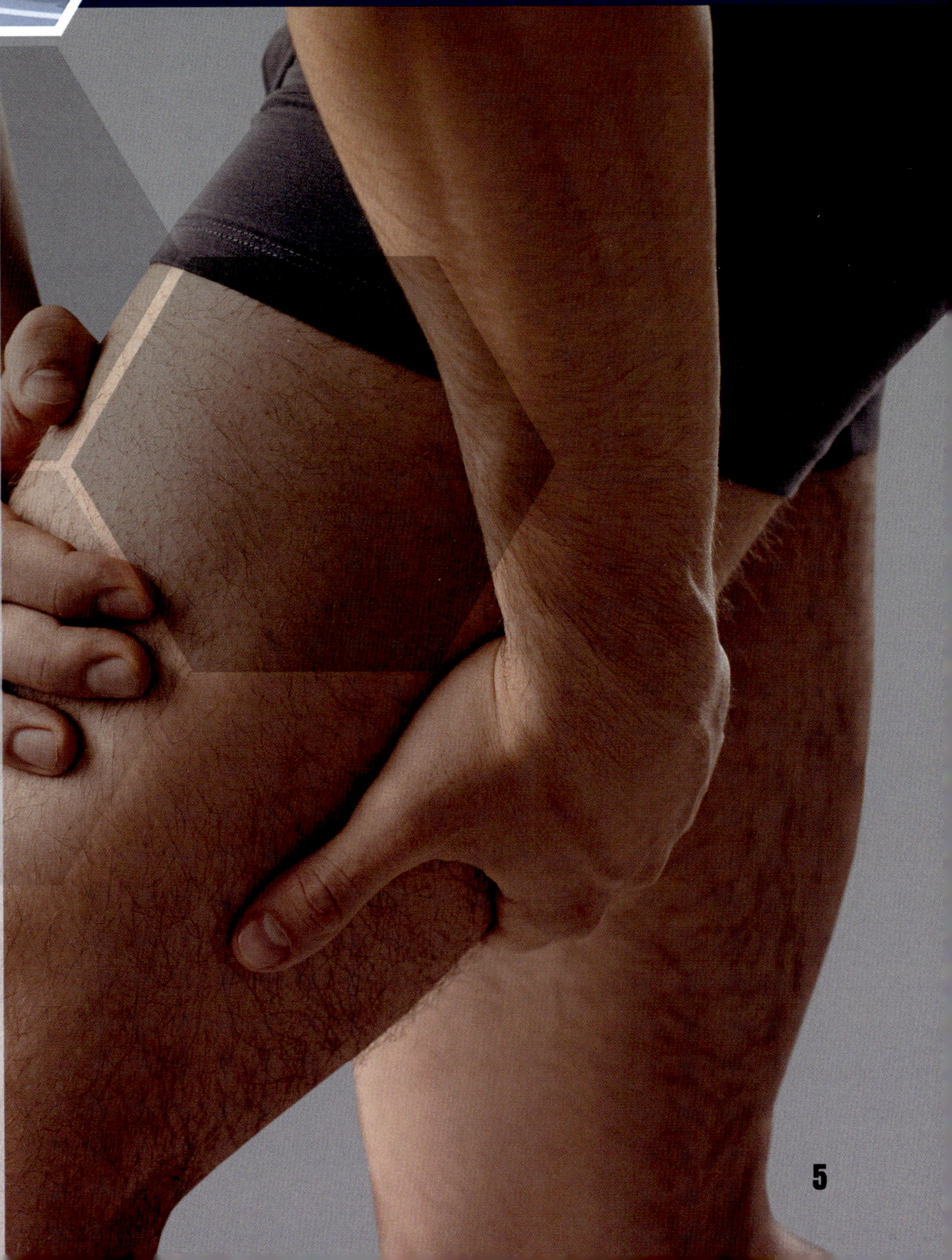

The name "hamstring" comes from two words. The first, "hamm," means "bend of the knee" in Old English. The second, "string," means tendon or ligament in Old English. Putting these two words together indicated the group of tendons or ligaments used to bend the knee. Today we use the word "hamstring" to refer to muscles, rather than tendons or ligaments.

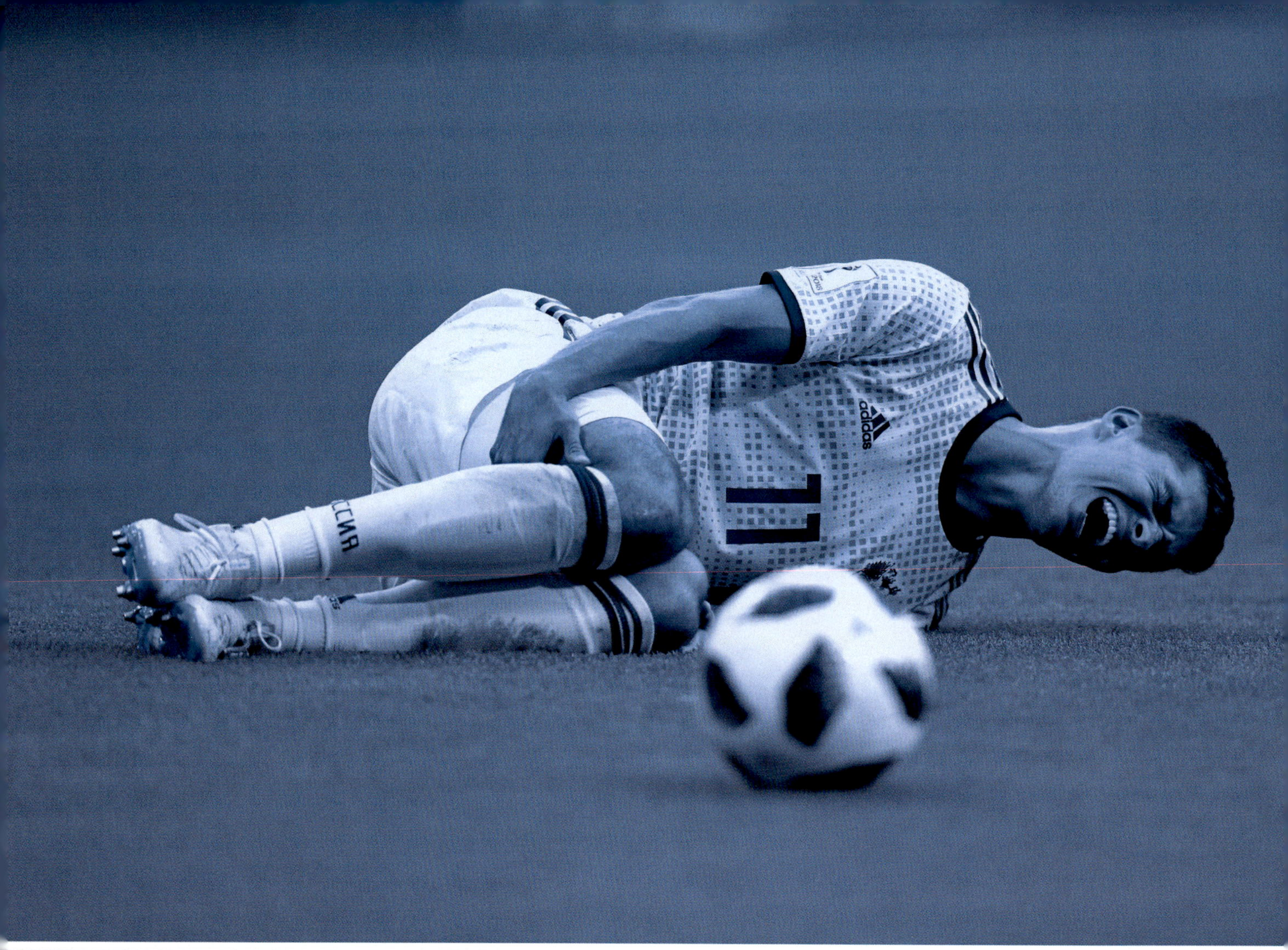

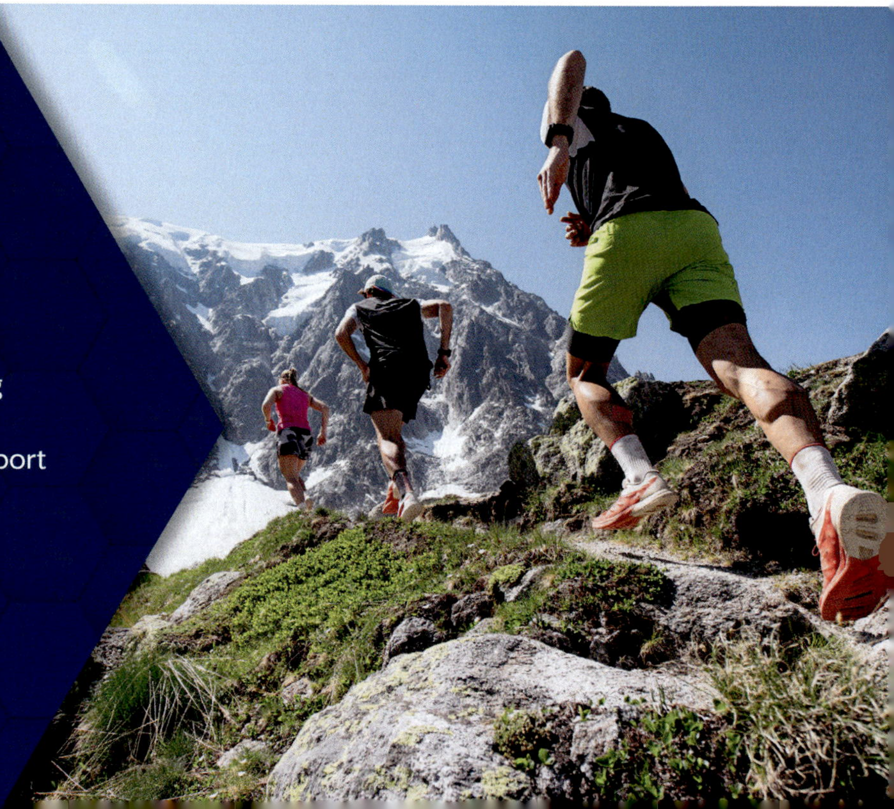

Hamstring injuries are a common way to get hurt while playing sports. Studies have found that almost a quarter of professional soccer players – both men and women – will lose playing time while recovering from hamstring injuries. But these injuries don't just affect soccer players. Players of any sport that involves running can hurt their hamstrings.

Fortunately, there are many ways to lower the chances of getting a hamstring injury. Doctors and physical therapists understand how to treat these injuries, and how to help players recover. You can help prevent hamstring injuries by learning how they happen.

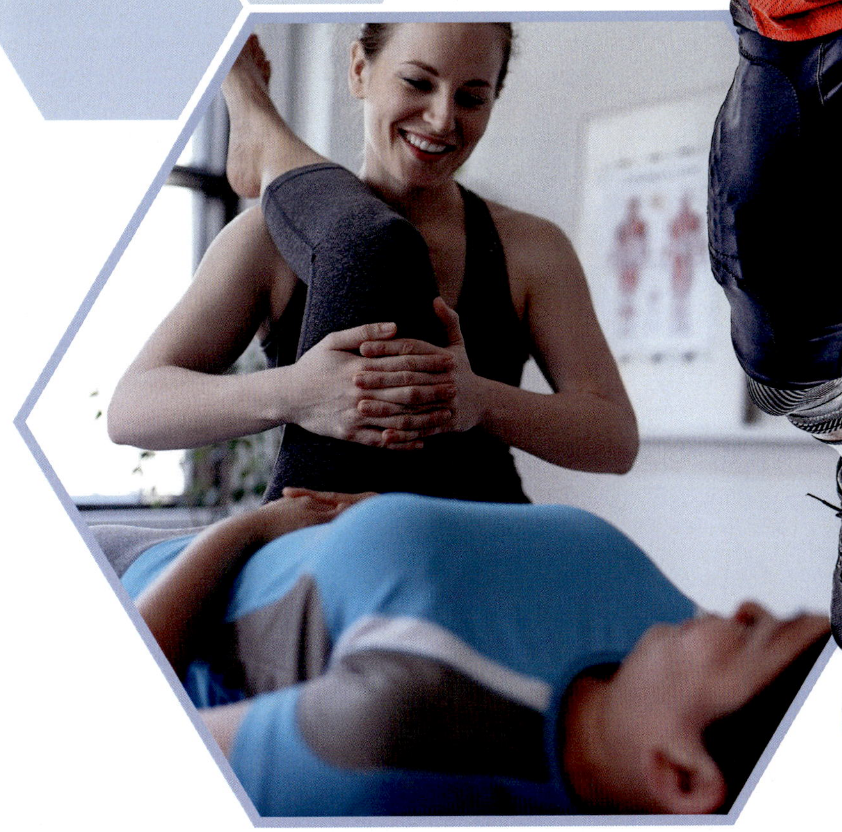

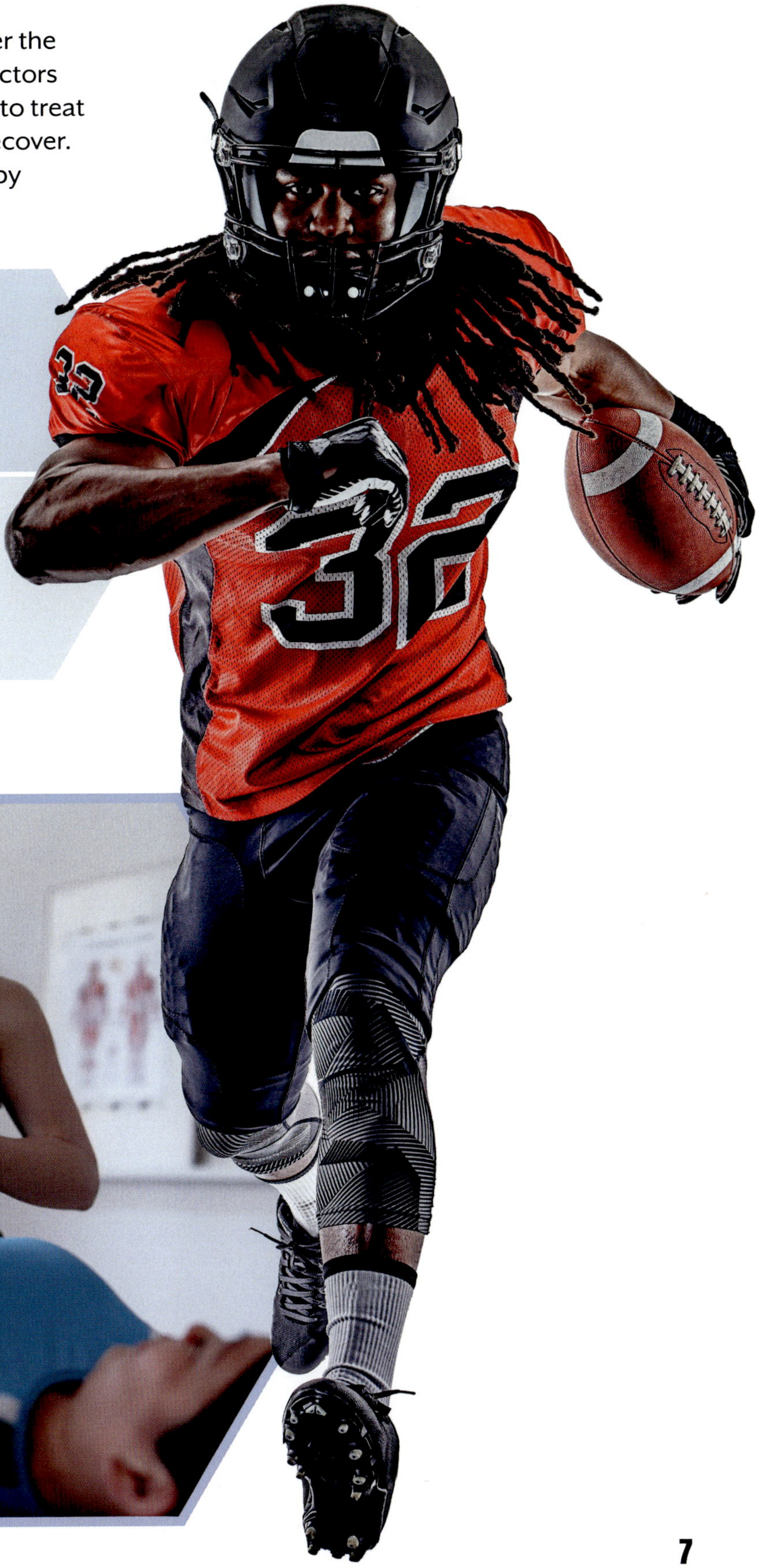

Chapter 2: Anatomy

Anatomy is a description of body parts and how they work together. Knowing the names, locations, and functions of **muscles**, **bones**, and **ligaments** is important in understanding how injuries happen.

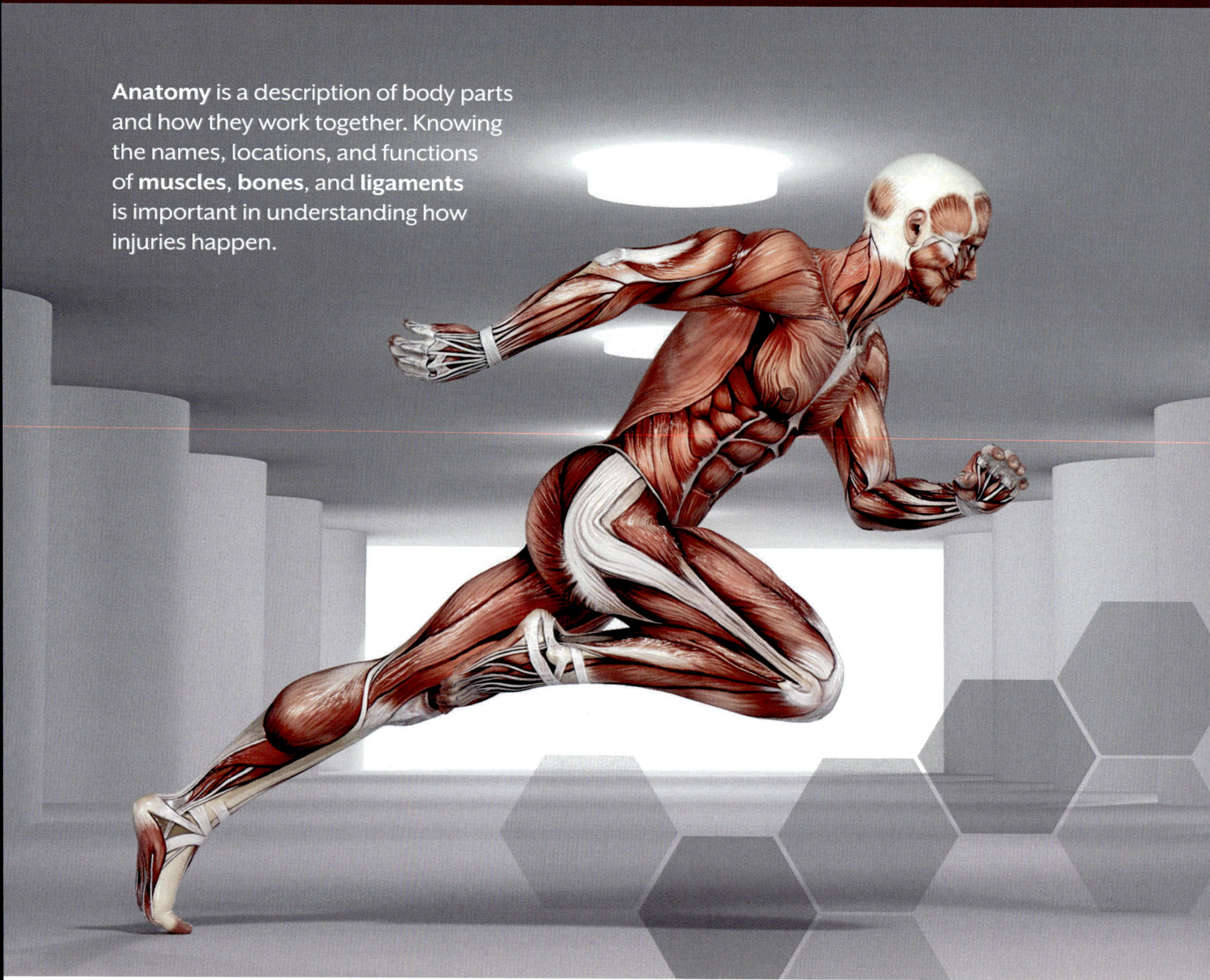

Bones and Muscles

The hamstrings are actually a group of three muscles.

The **pelvis** is a group of bones that make up your lower torso, commonly known as the hip bones. The **tibia**, or shin bone, is the long bone of your lower leg. The **semimembranosus** and **semitendinosus** are two muscles that run from your pelvis to the inside of your tibia. The semimembranosus muscle is thinner than the semitendinosus muscle, but they are located next to each other.

The **biceps femoris** is a muscle that starts in two places. One part of the biceps femoris begins on your pelvis. This is called the long head. The other part of the biceps femoris begins on your **femur**, or the long bone of the upper leg. This is called the short head. Both parts of the biceps femoris combine into one muscle. This muscle ends on the fibula, which is a smaller bone next to the tibia.

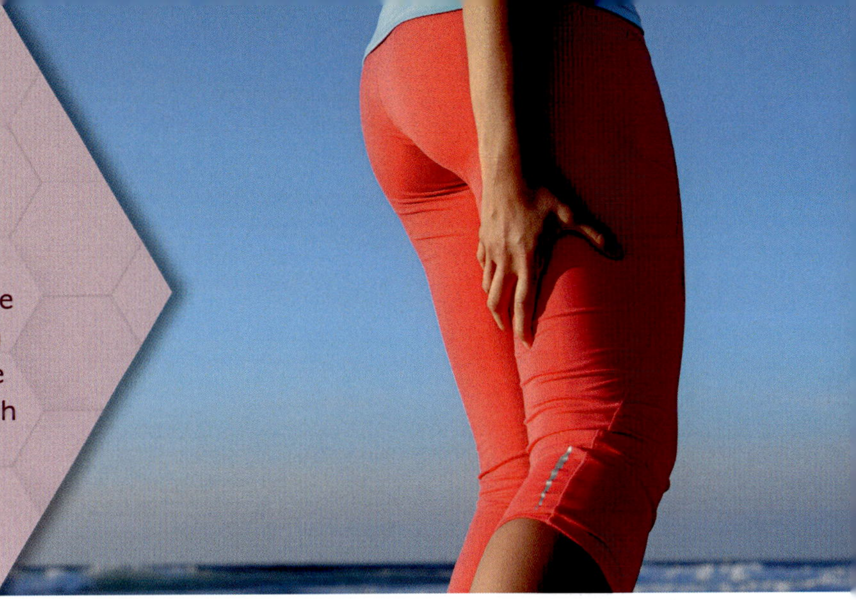

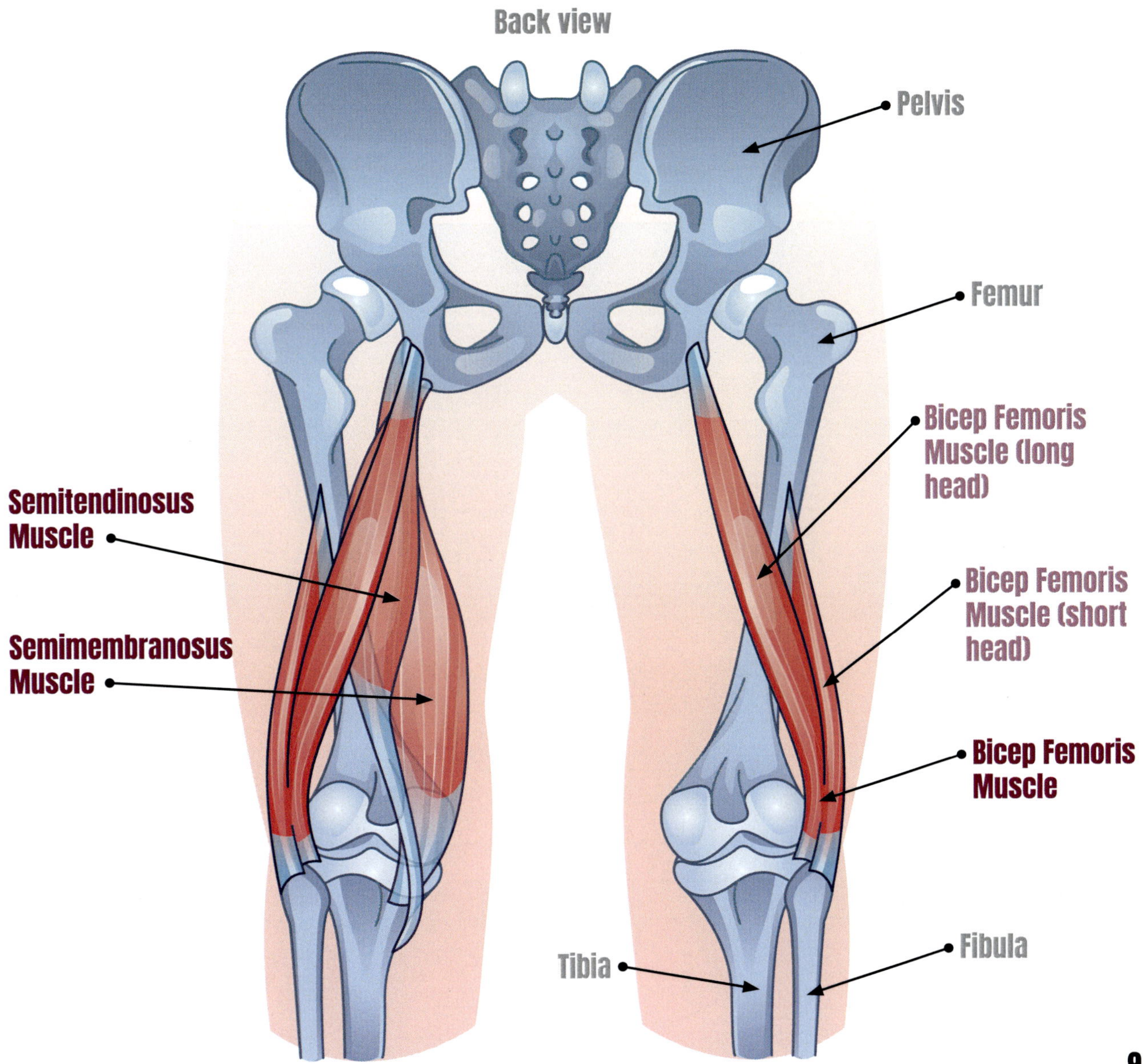

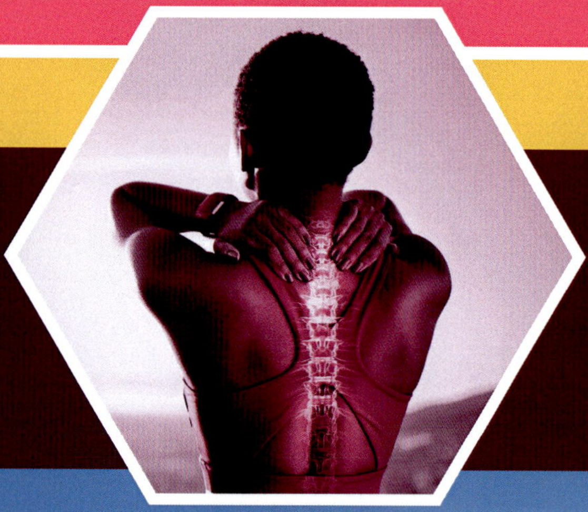

Joints

The place where two or more bones come together is called a **joint**. Some joints, such as the bones of your skull, don't move. Other joints, such as the bones of your spine, move just a little bit. However, many joints in your body move a lot. These are called **mobile joints**.

The hamstrings muscles cross over two joints: your hip joint and your knee joint. Both the hip and the knees are mobile joints. Your hip joint connects your pelvis and your femur. Your hip joint helps support your upper body while you walk and run. It also helps to keep your body balanced while you move. Your knee joint connects your femur to your tibia. Like your hip joint, your knees help support your body. They let your legs swing during movement.

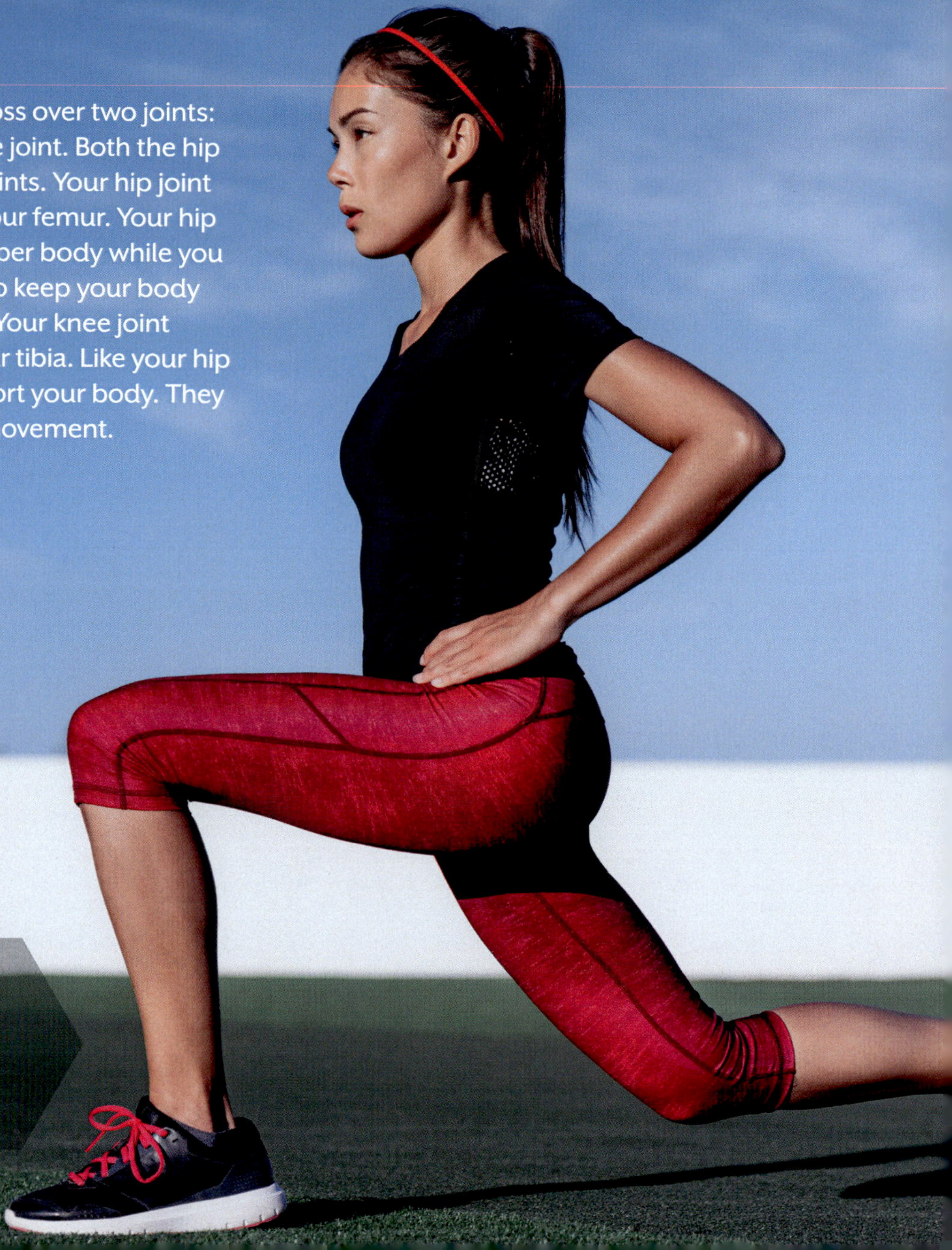

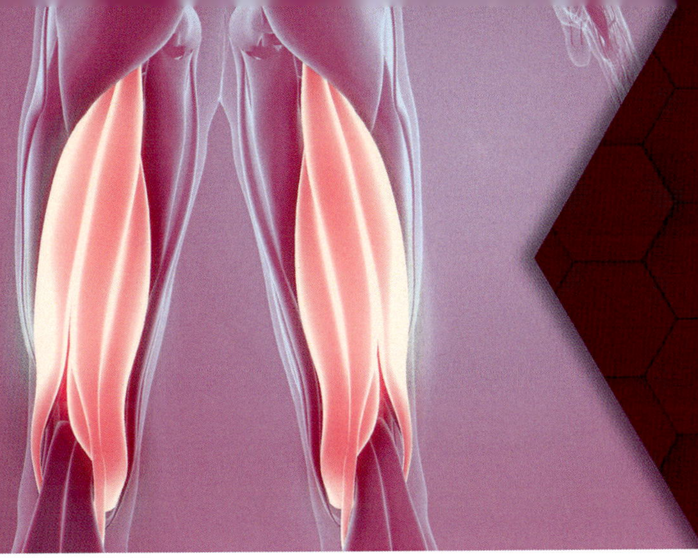

The muscles of your hamstrings are responsible for three motions:

- Bending the knee joint
- Extending the hip joint
- Rotating the hip joint

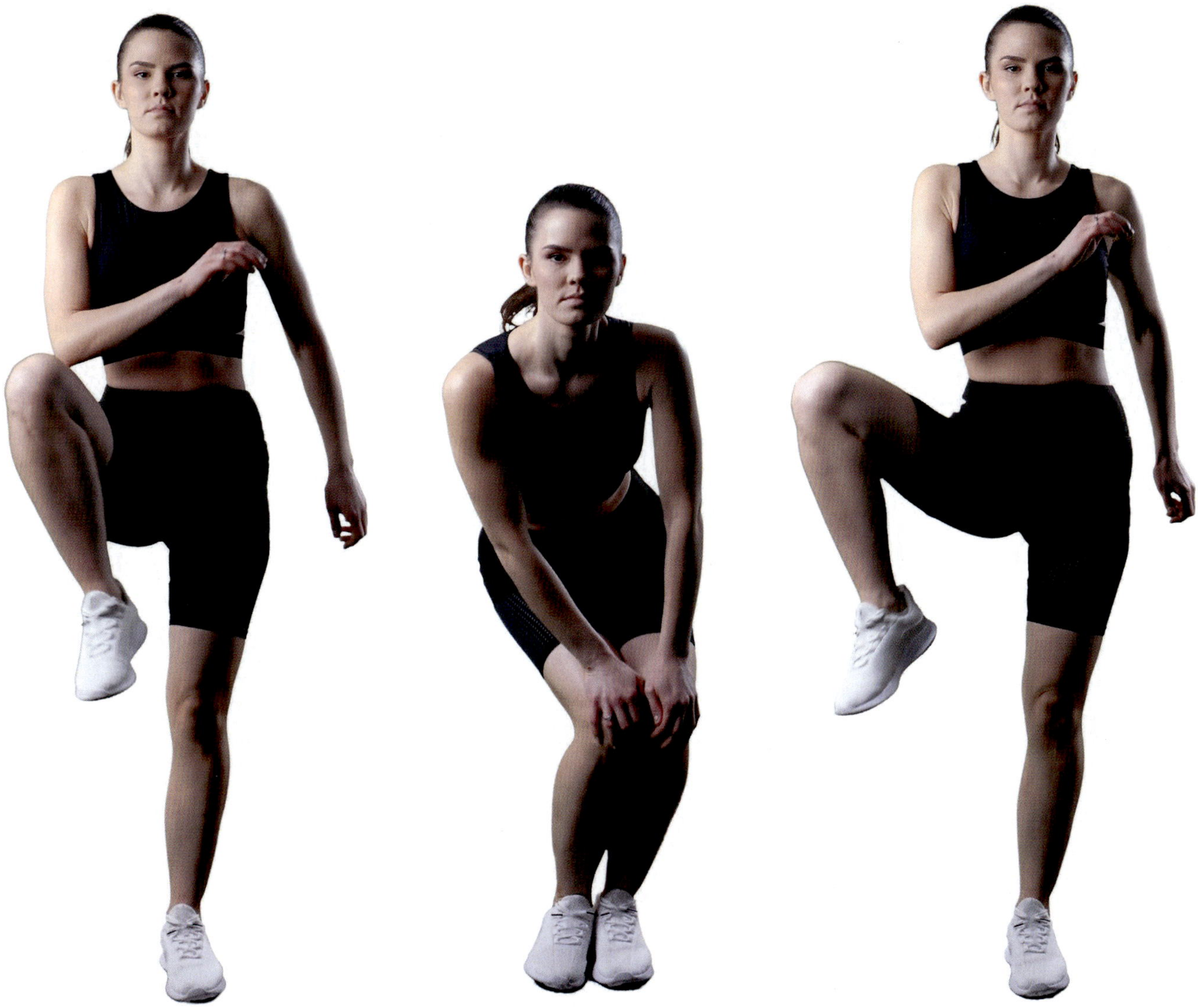

Sometimes people use the words "tendon" and "ligament" to mean the same thing, but they're actually different. Tendons connect muscle to bone. Ligaments connect bones to other bones.

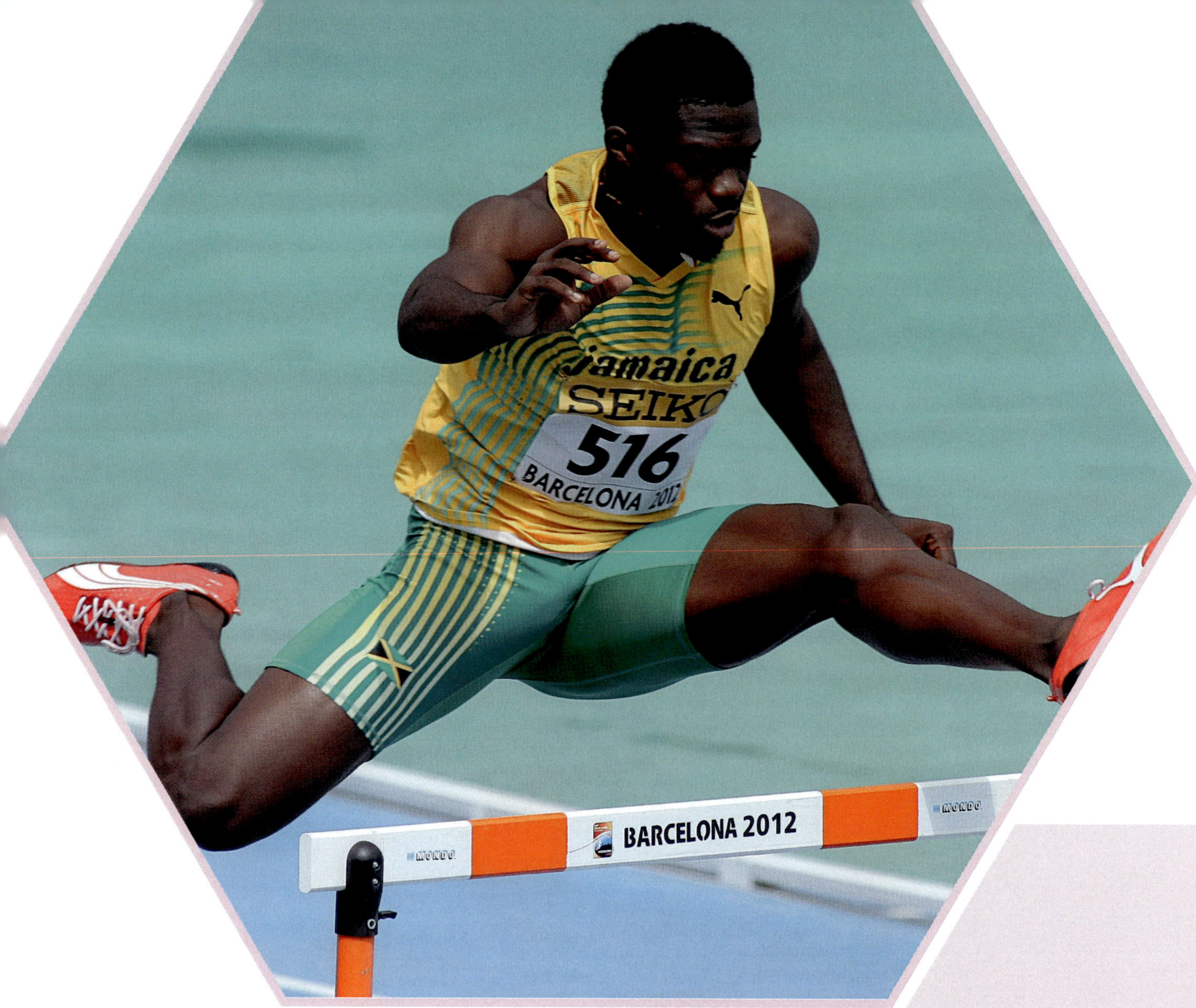

When you bend your knee, your hamstrings pull your lower leg closer to your upper leg. Bending the knee means that the hamstrings help bring the lower leg closer to the upper leg. When you extend your hip joint, your hamstrings move your upper leg backward. Your hamstring muscles also help with hip rotation by moving your leg in both clockwise and counterclockwise motions.

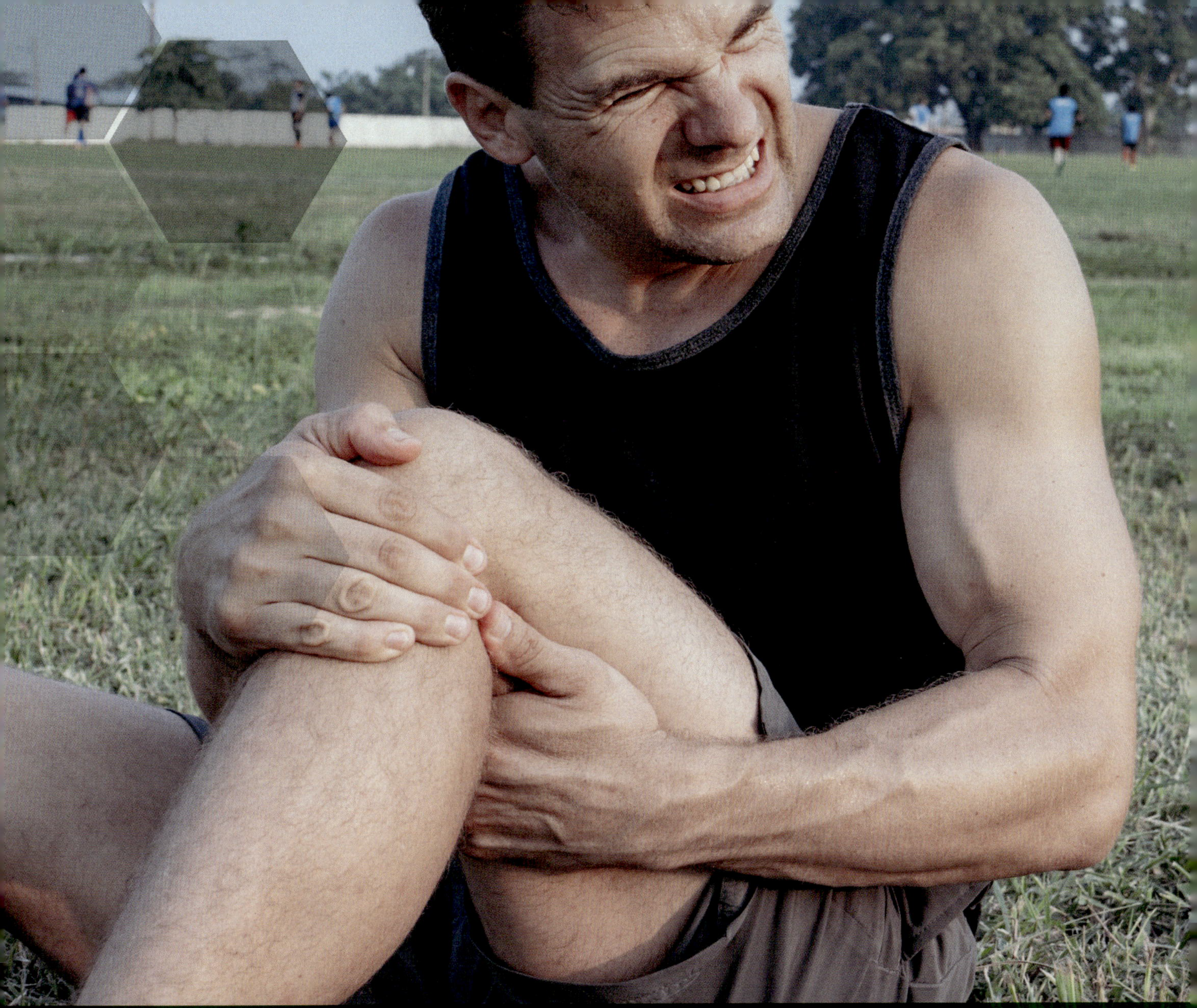

Chapter 3: Causes of Hamstring Injuries

Hamstring injuries happen when one or more of the hamstring muscles are stretched too far. These are **acute injuries**. That means they happen suddenly.

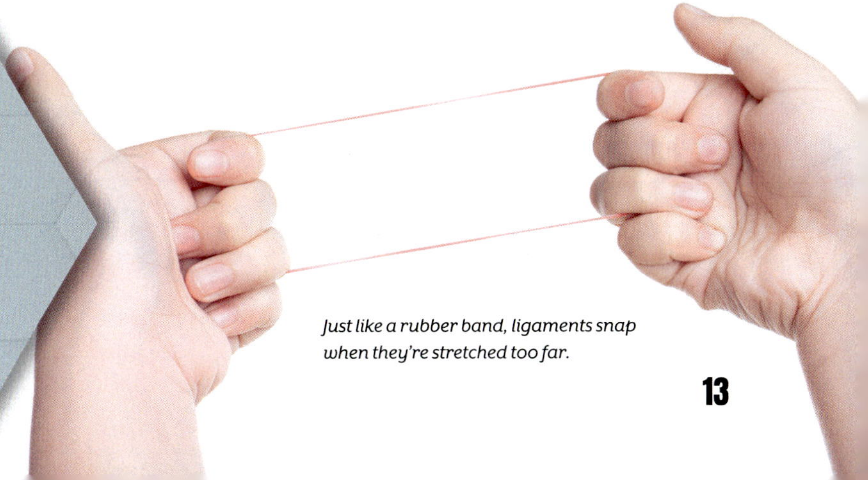

Just like a rubber band, ligaments snap when they're stretched too far.

Tendons are soft tissue that connect your muscle to bone. Many hamstring injuries occur where muscle and tendon meet. Other hamstring injuries happen where tendon attaches to bone.

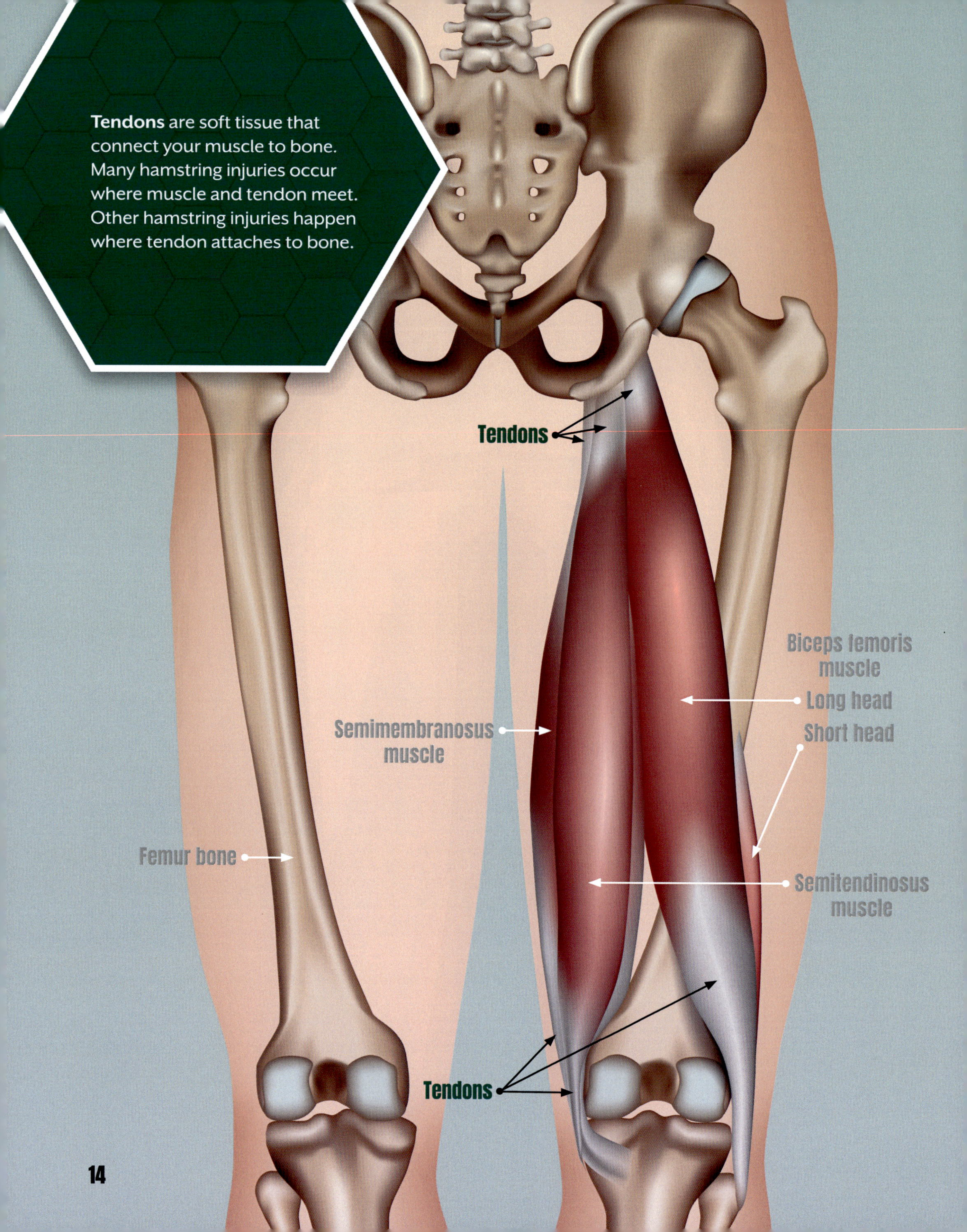

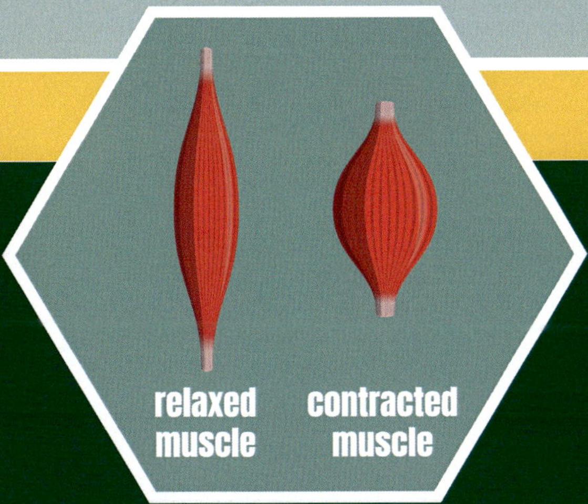

Contraction

Muscles move bones by contracting, or getting smaller. When the muscle fibers pull against one another, the muscle gets shorter. As the muscle contracts, bones are brought closer together. Think about your knee joint. When you kick your heel toward the back of your thigh, the bones of your lower leg are brought closer to your upper leg. This motion is because your hamstring muscles have worked by contracting across the knee joint.

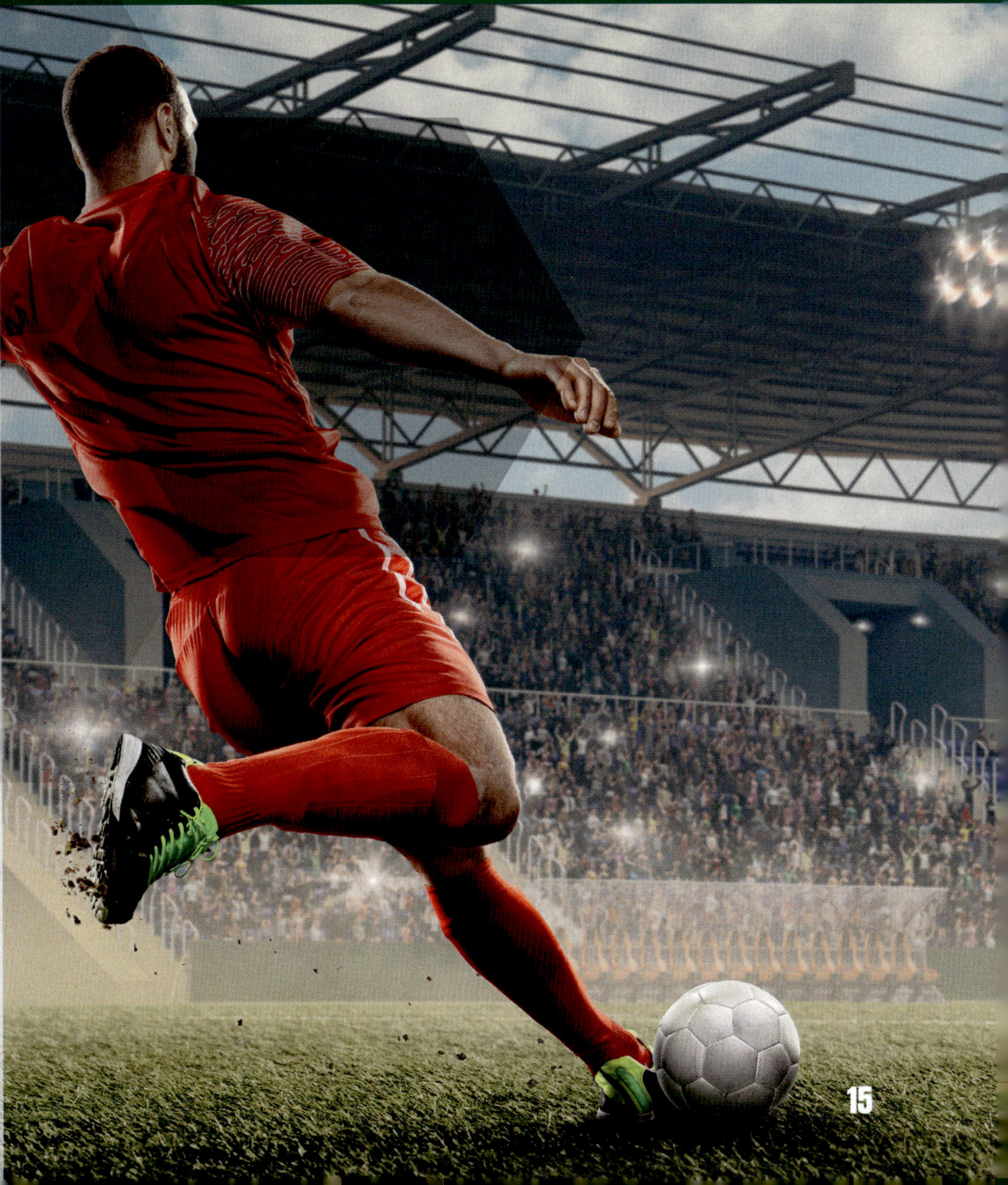

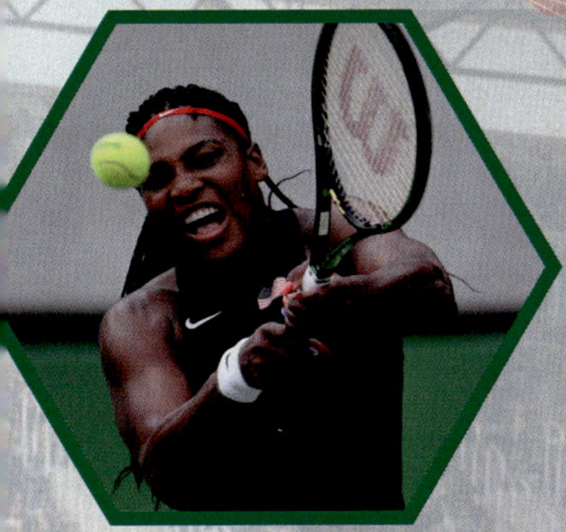

Many famous athletes have had hamstring injuries. David Beckham, Kobe Bryant, Usain Bolt, Tiger Woods, Serena Williams, and LeBron James have all had this injury.

Eccentric Contraction

There are times when a muscle needs to contract while also lengthening. These are called **eccentric contractions**. When a runner's front leg is reaching to the ground, her hamstring muscles are in eccentric contraction. The hamstring muscles contract to slow the runner's leg and control its speed while also getting longer as her leg stretches forward.

This combination of muscle contraction while lengthening may lead to injury because of the high forces in the muscle during this motion.

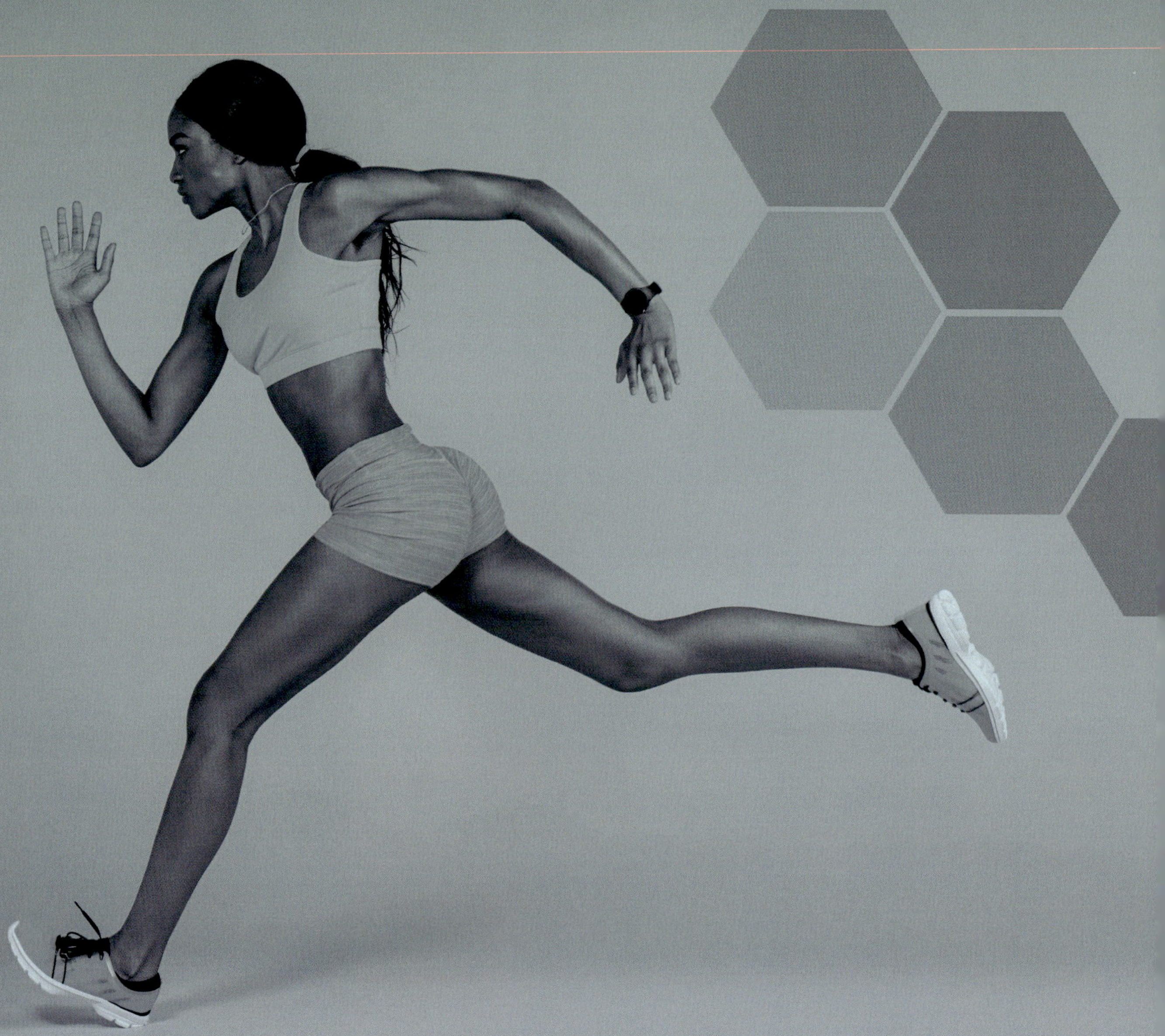

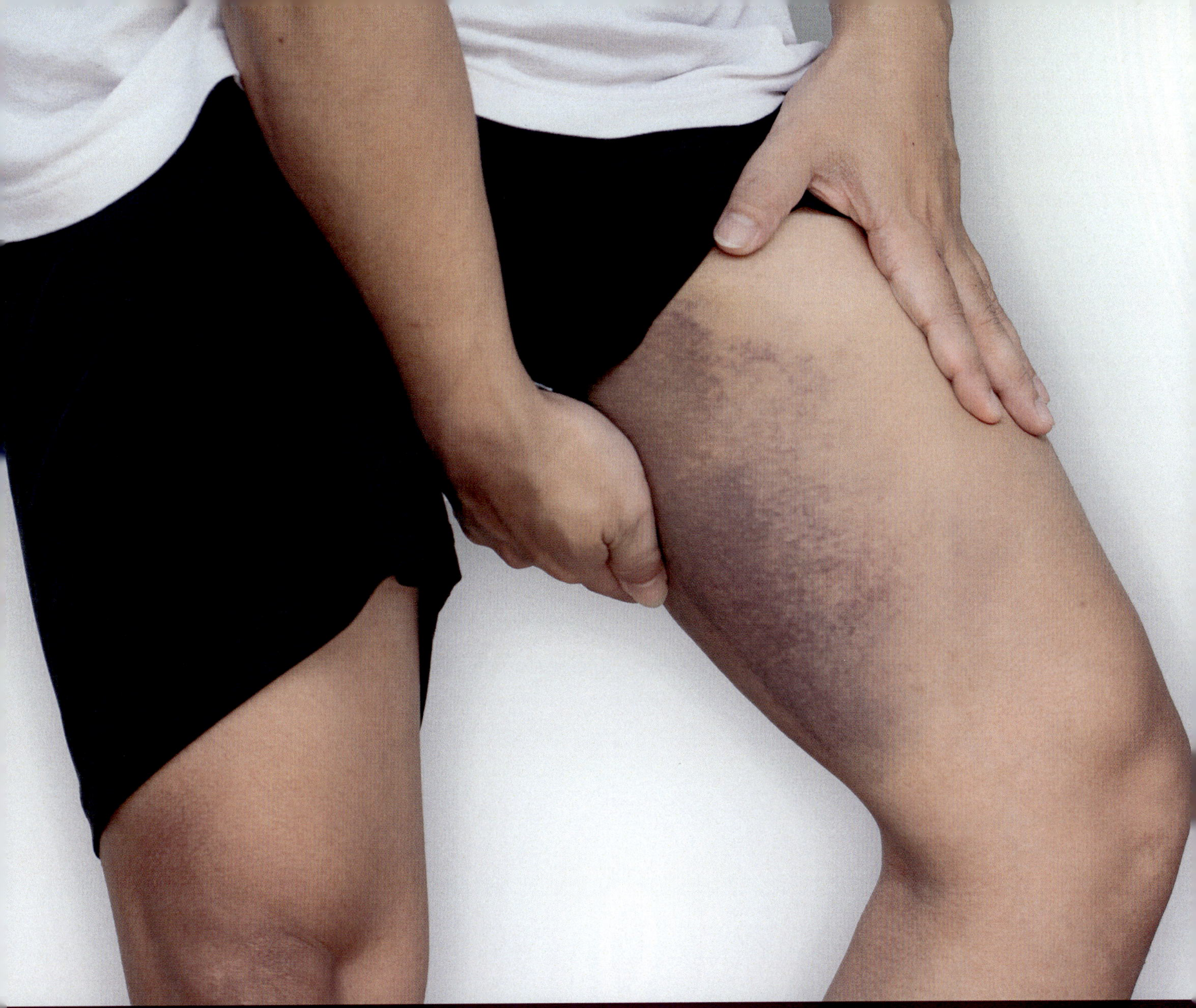

Chapter 4: Types of Hamstring Injuries

Many athletes have hamstring injuries. These injuries can range from just a small muscle strain to a complete tear. Doctors and medical professionals developed a grading system to help identify the types of injury. They use this grading system to recommend treatment.

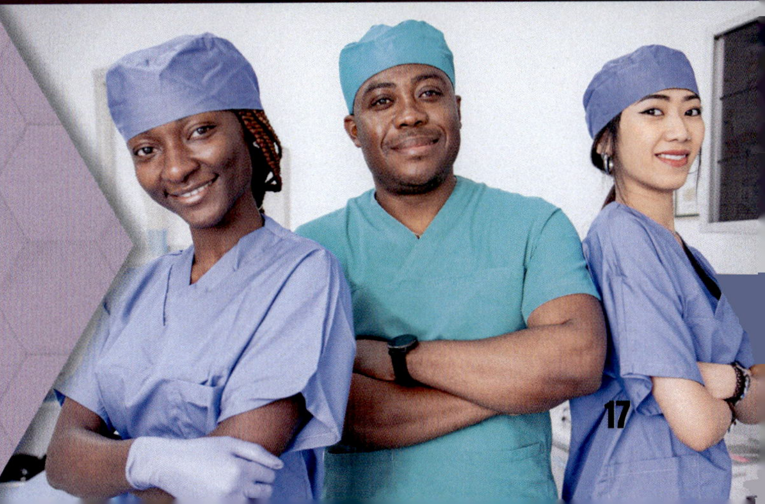

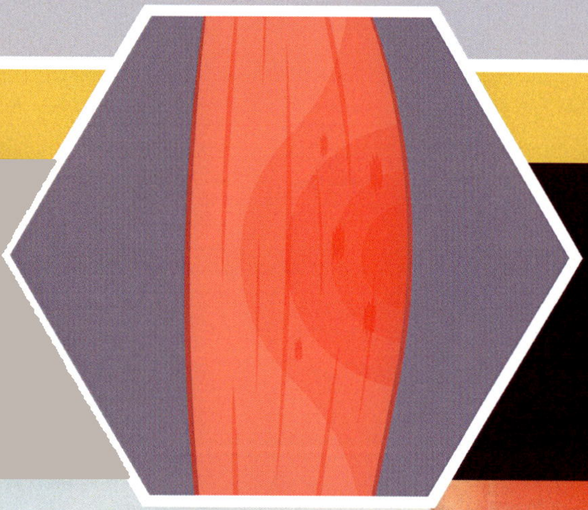

Grade 1

Grade 1 hamstring injuries are the least severe. Athletes who have a Grade 1 injury have a mild pulled muscle or strain. They may only have a slight loss of strength in the muscle, and they will only notice a slight of change in the **range of motion** of their legs.

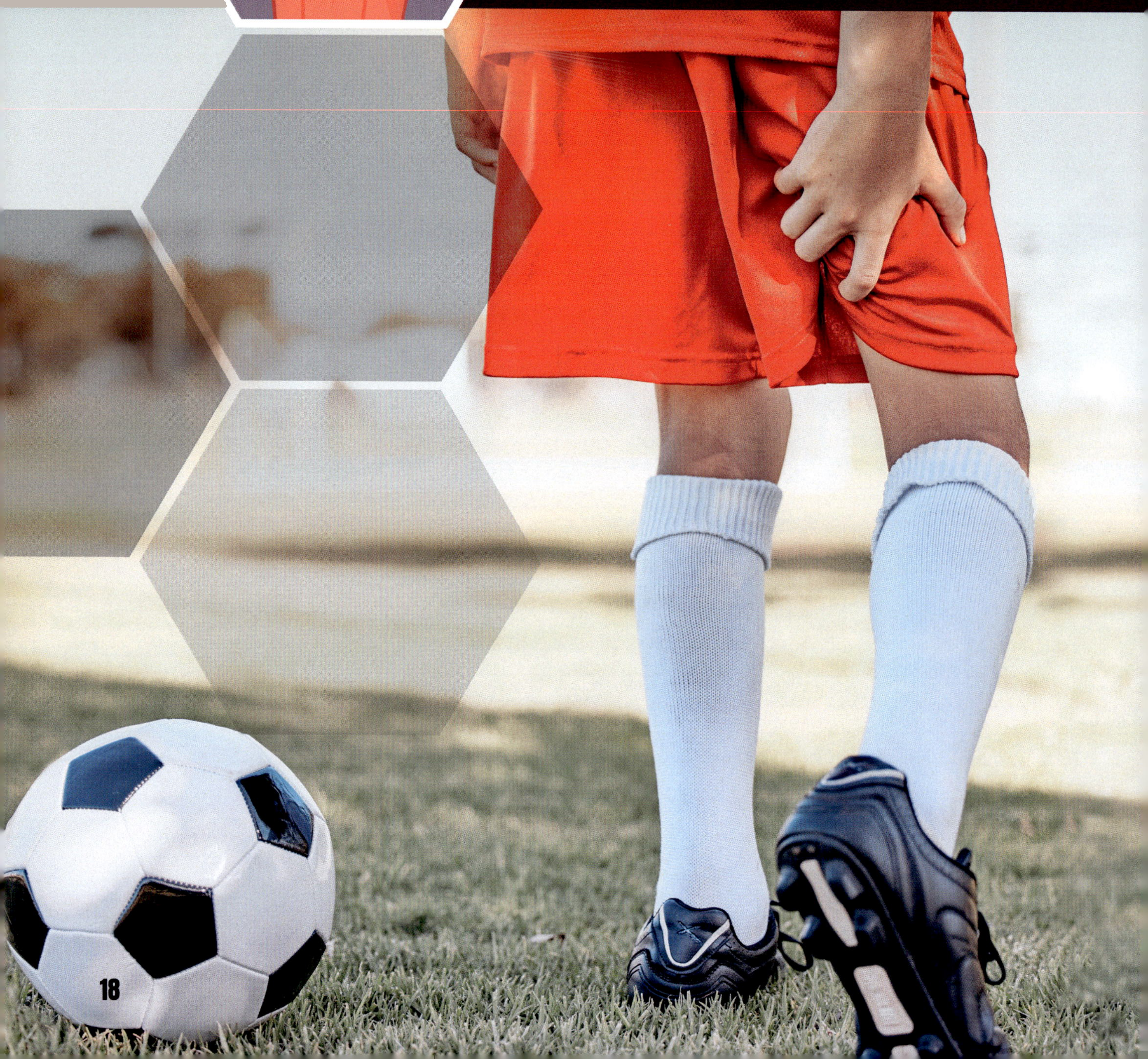

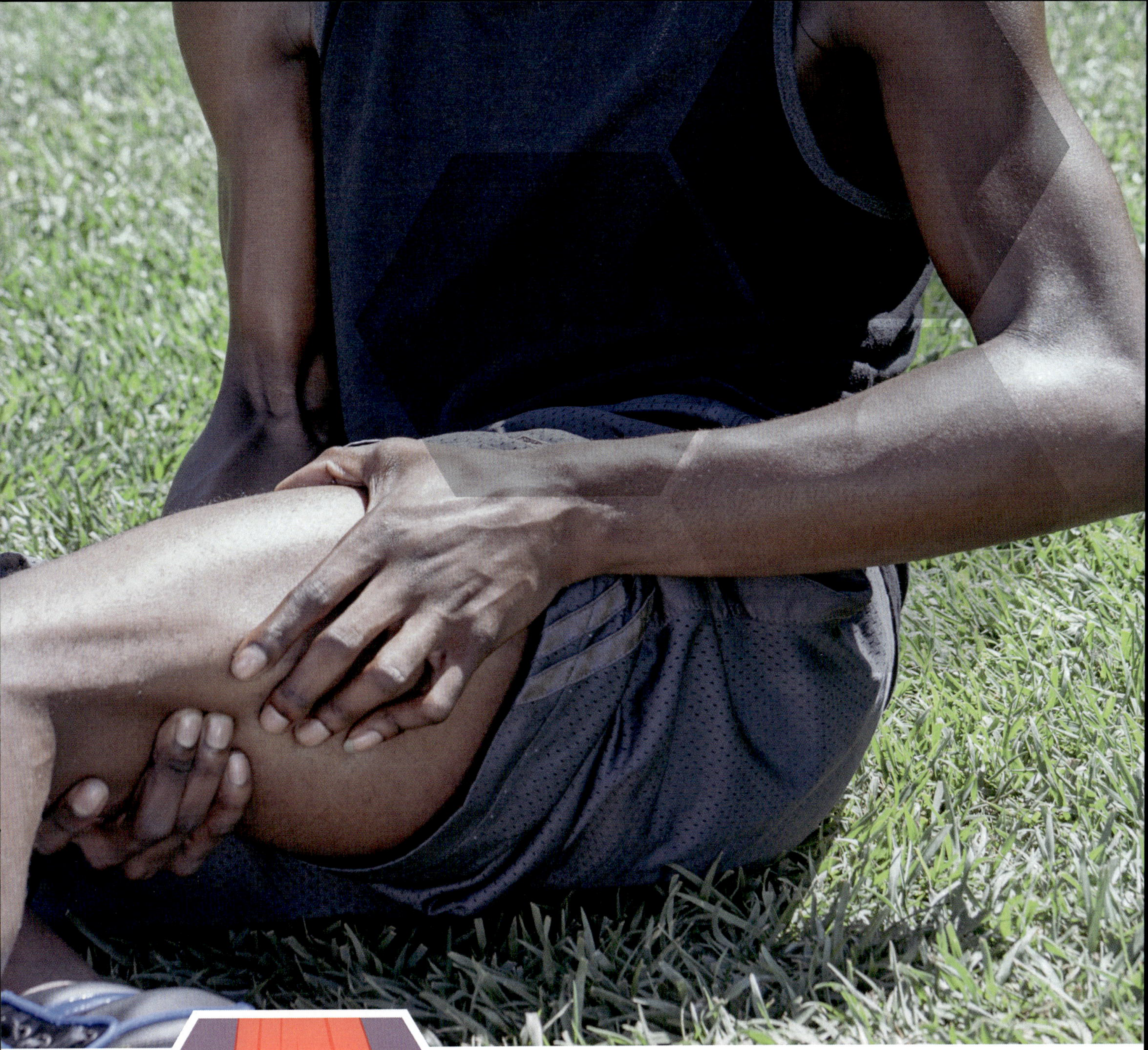

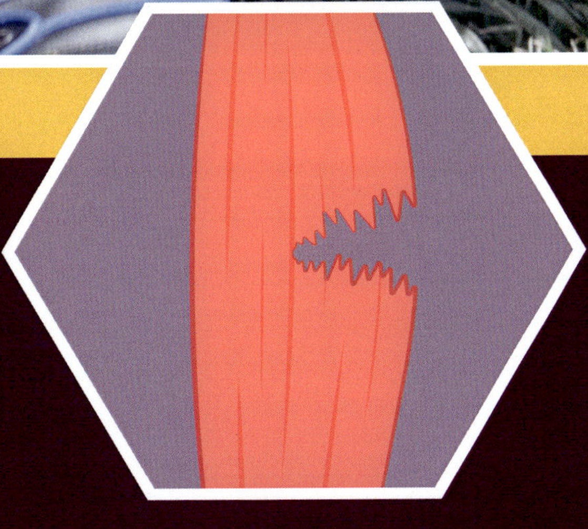

Grade 2

Athletes with a Grade 2 hamstring injury have a partial tear of the muscle or tendon. This partial tear may cause an athlete to limp or have trouble walking. There is usually some loss of range of motion with this injury, which means that an athlete may not be able to fully straighten their leg. The athlete's leg may also swell and bruise in a Grade 2 hamstring injury.

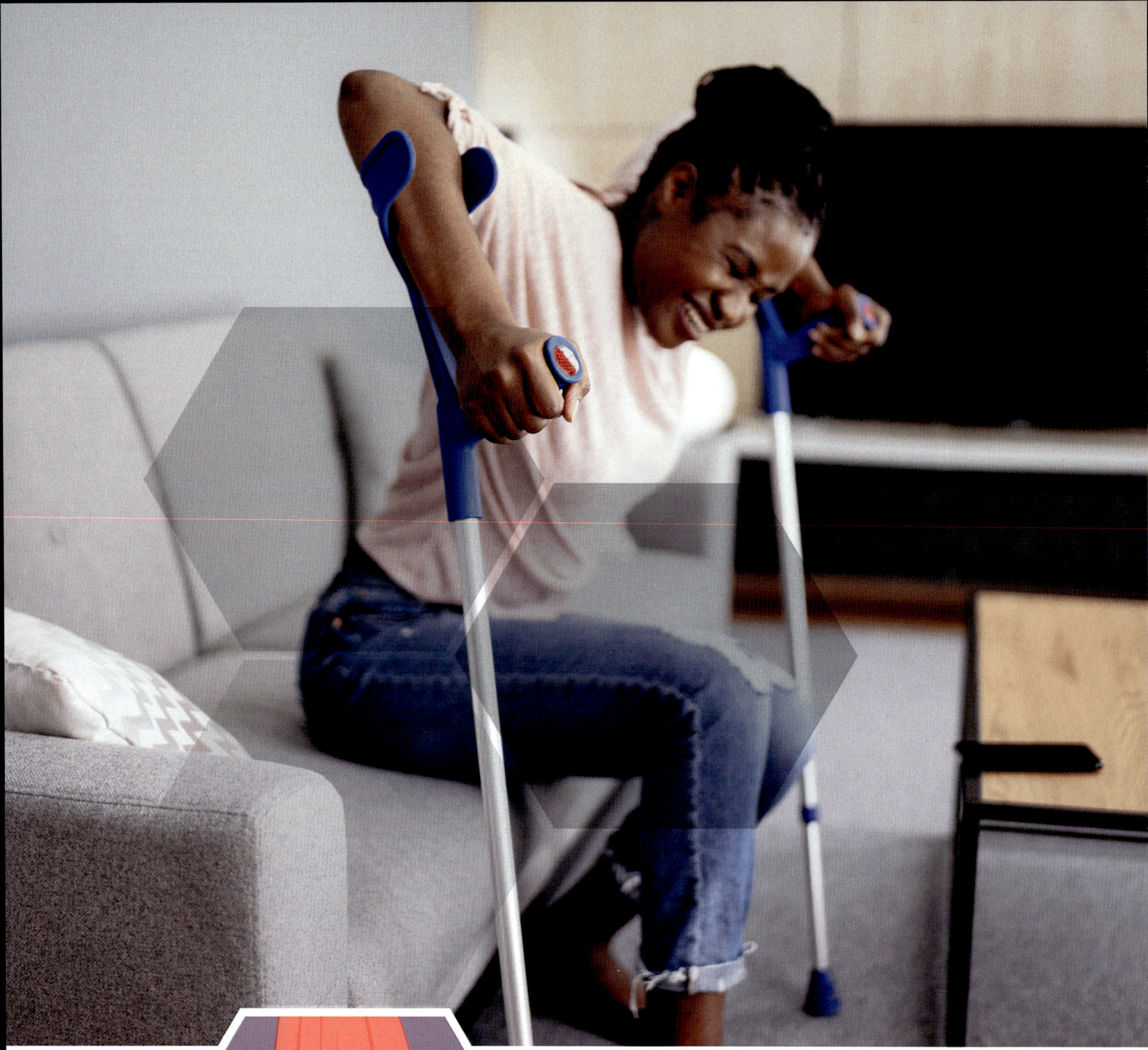

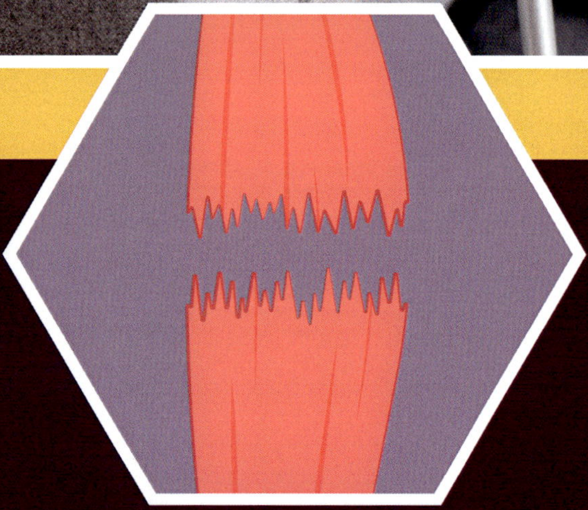

Grade 3

Grade 3 hamstring injuries are the most severe. These injuries have a full tear of the muscle or tendon. Athletes will not be able to fully straighten their leg, and the muscle will be painful. Almost immediately after the injury occurs, there will be significant swelling and bruising. Even movement such as walking will be difficult, and the athlete may require crutches.

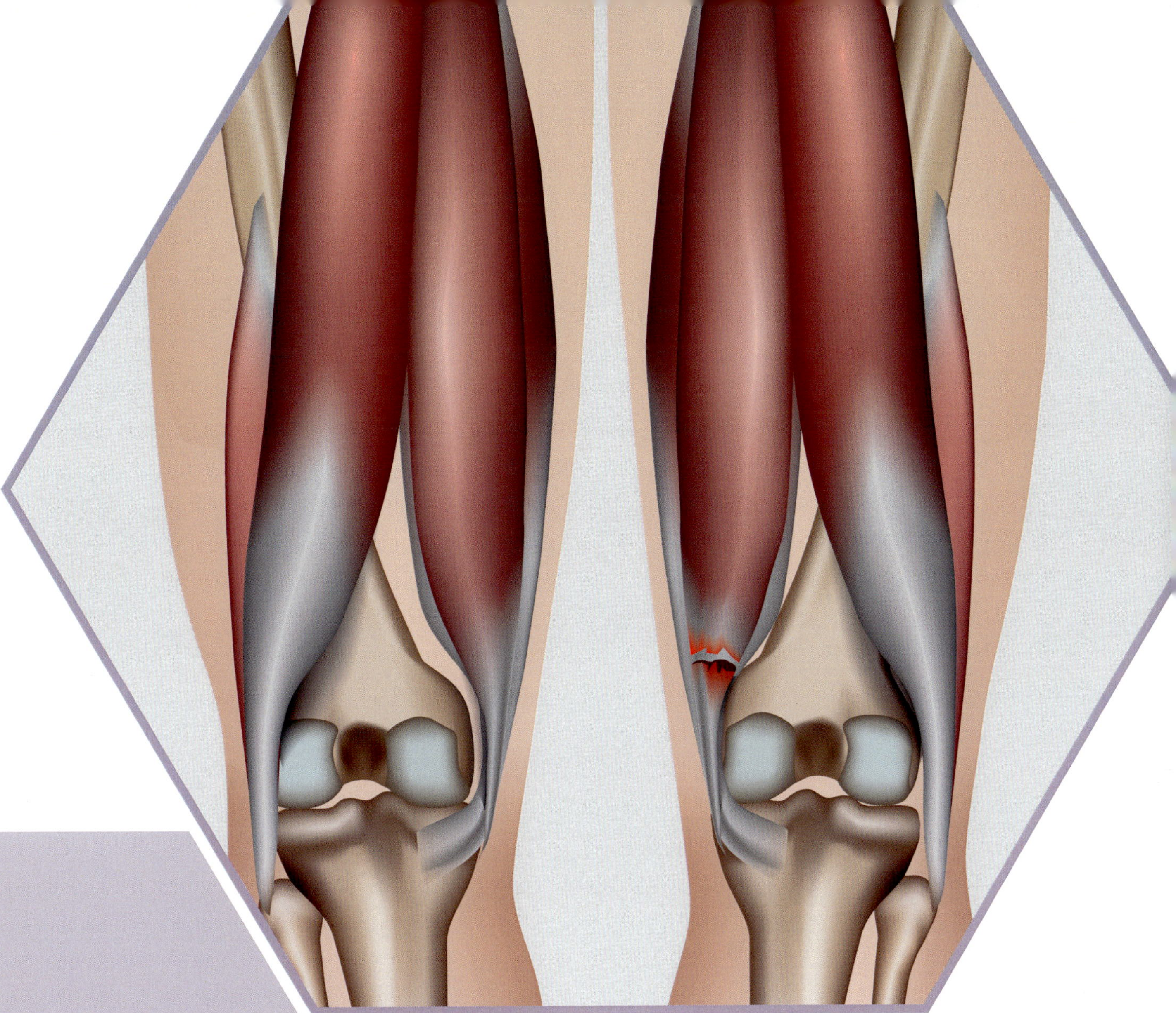

In most cases, tears occur in the thick part of one of the muscles or at the point where tendon and muscle meet. However, Grade 3 hamstring tears may also occur at the meeting point of the muscle tendon and bone. These are called **avulsion injuries**. Some avulsion injuries may even tear part of the bone away.

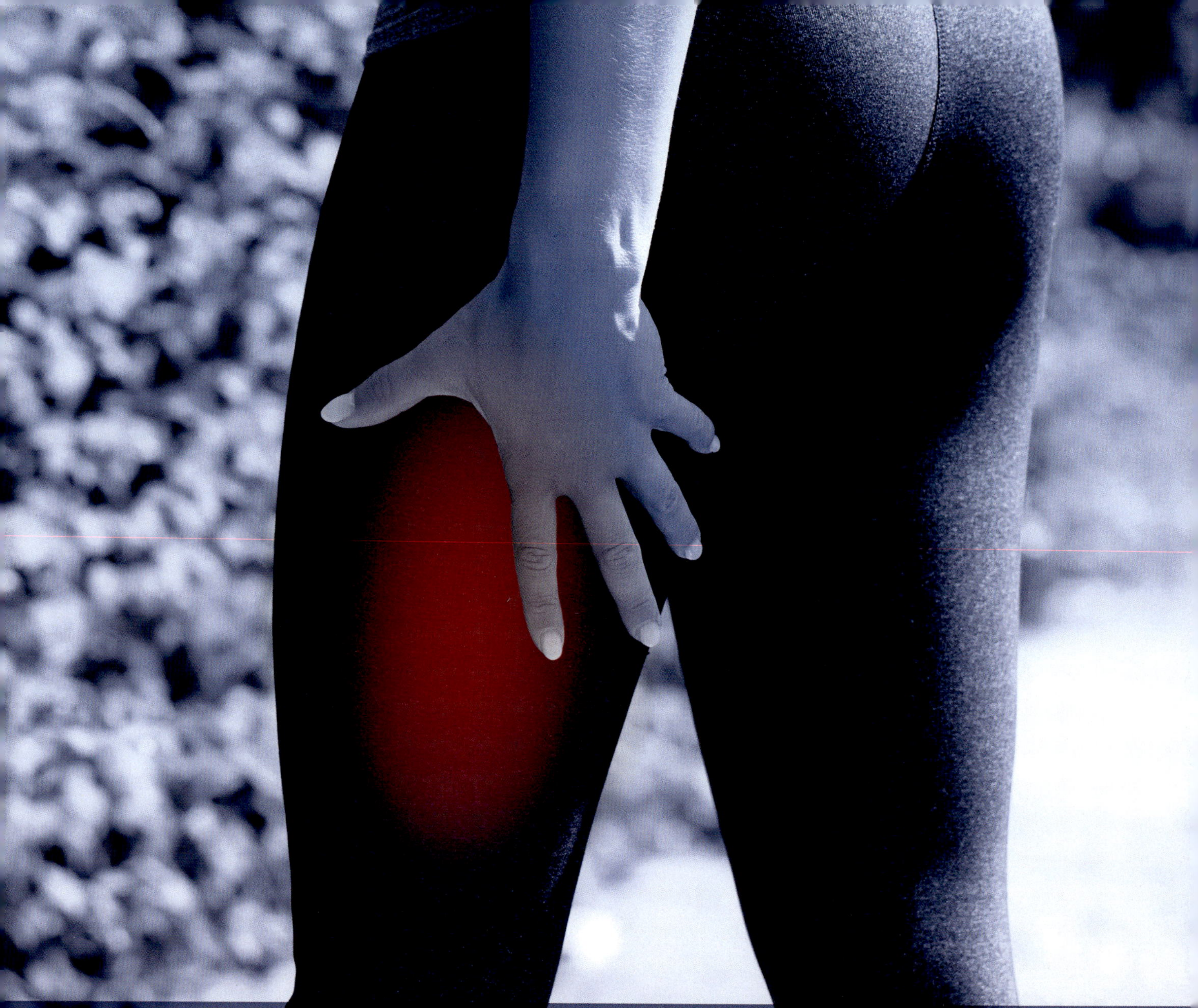

Chapter 5: Diagnosis

An athlete usually notices a hamstring injury while they are running. They feel a sharp pain in the back of one of their upper legs. The pain may be so bad that they have to stop running. They may fall to the ground or only be able to hop on their uninjured leg.

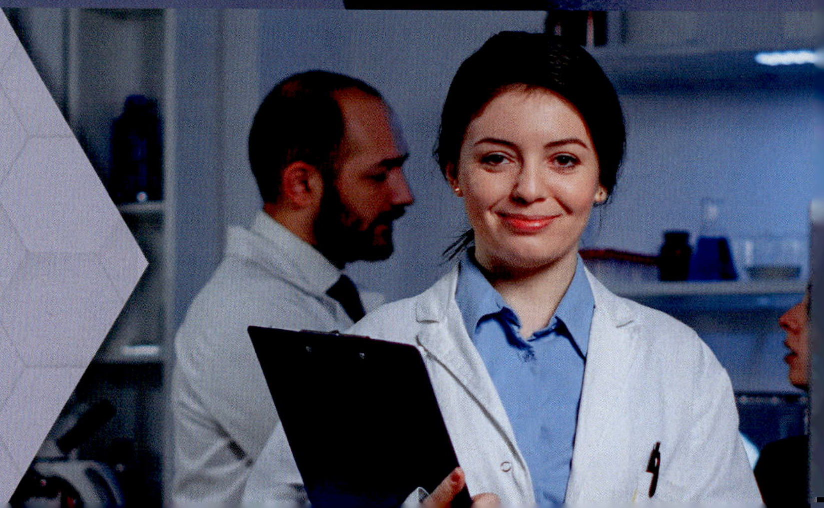

The athlete may notice other symptoms of injury. There may be swelling where the muscle has been torn. There also may be bruising around the injury site.

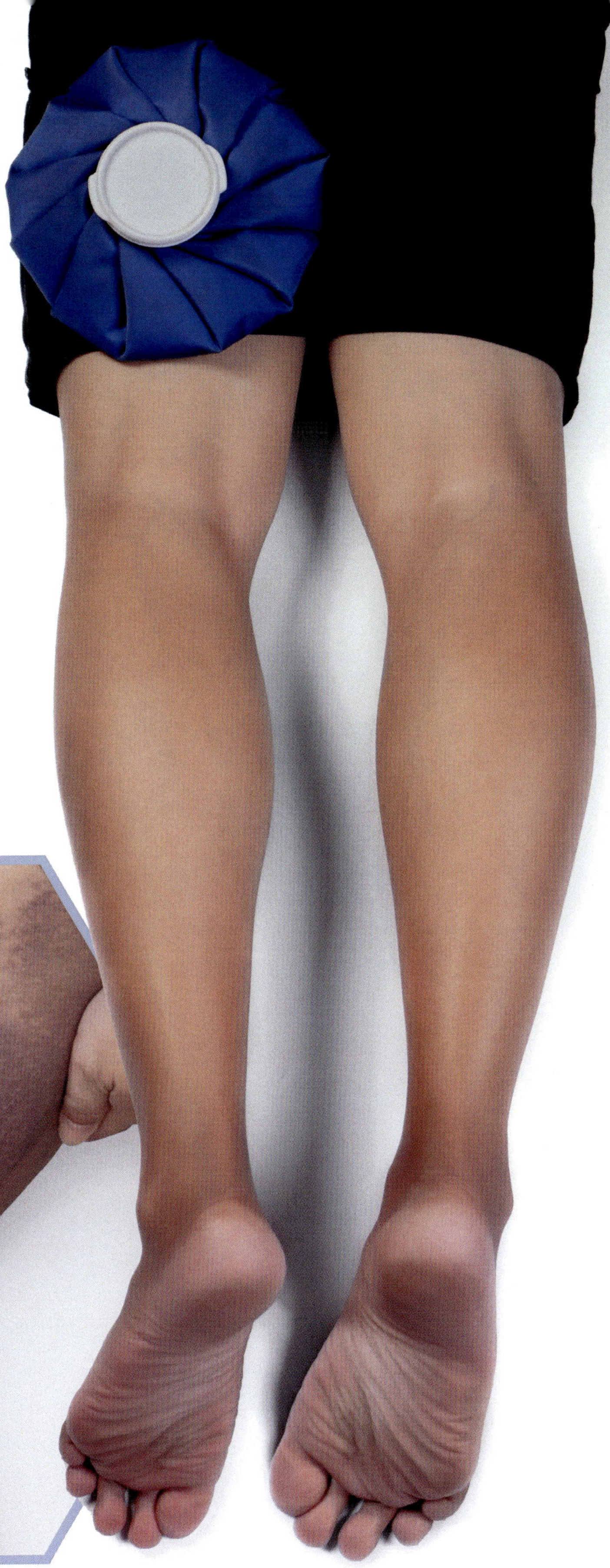

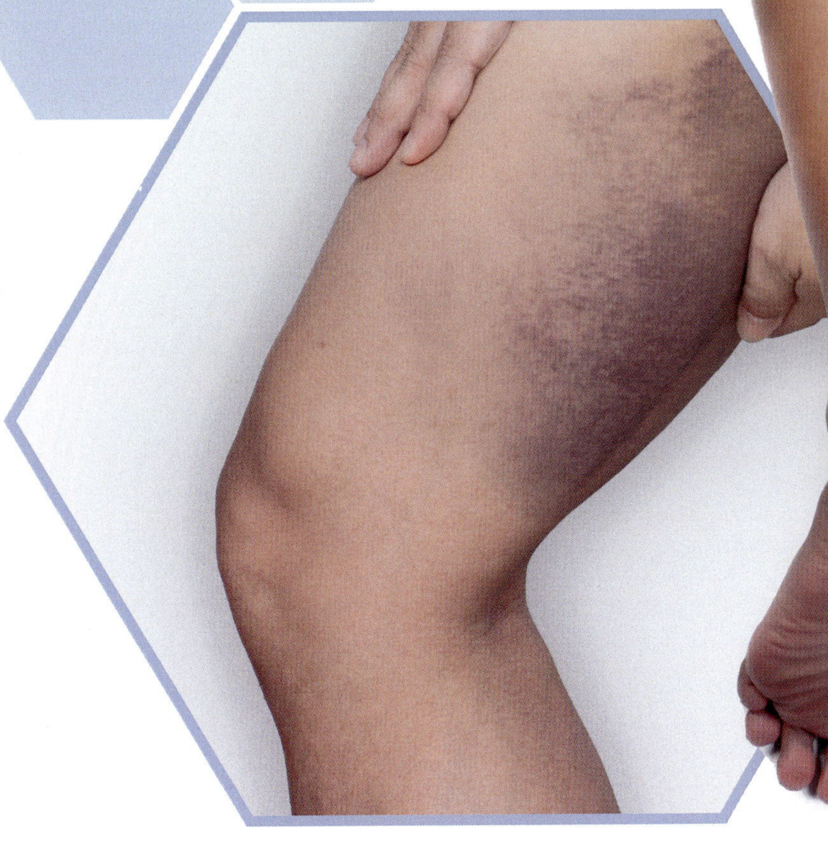

Medical Examination

Doctors and athletic trainers examine an injured athlete. They ask the athlete how the injury feels and what happened around the time they first felt pain.

The hamstring muscles receive signals from the brain along the sciatic nerve. This is the longest nerve in your body!

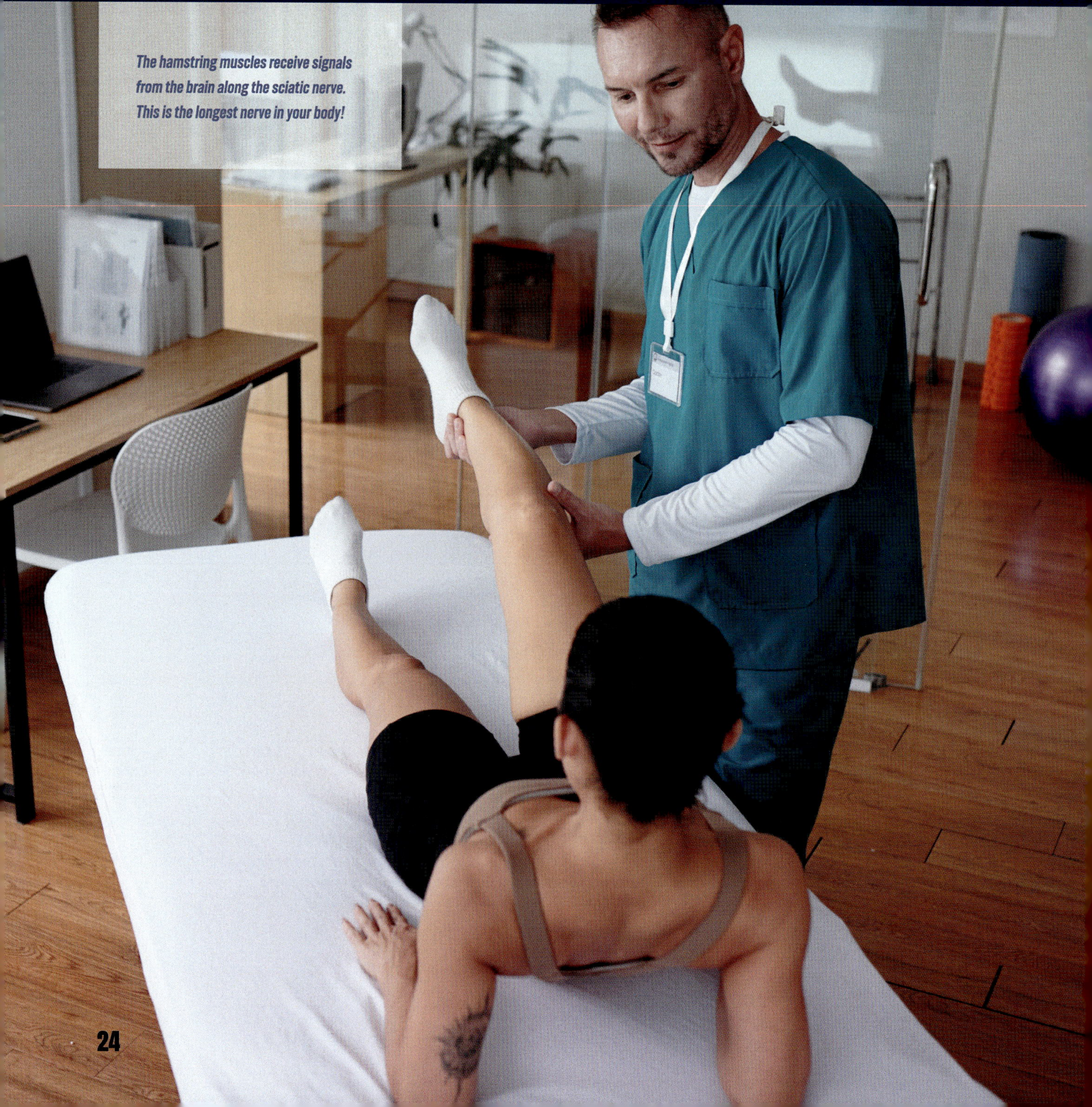

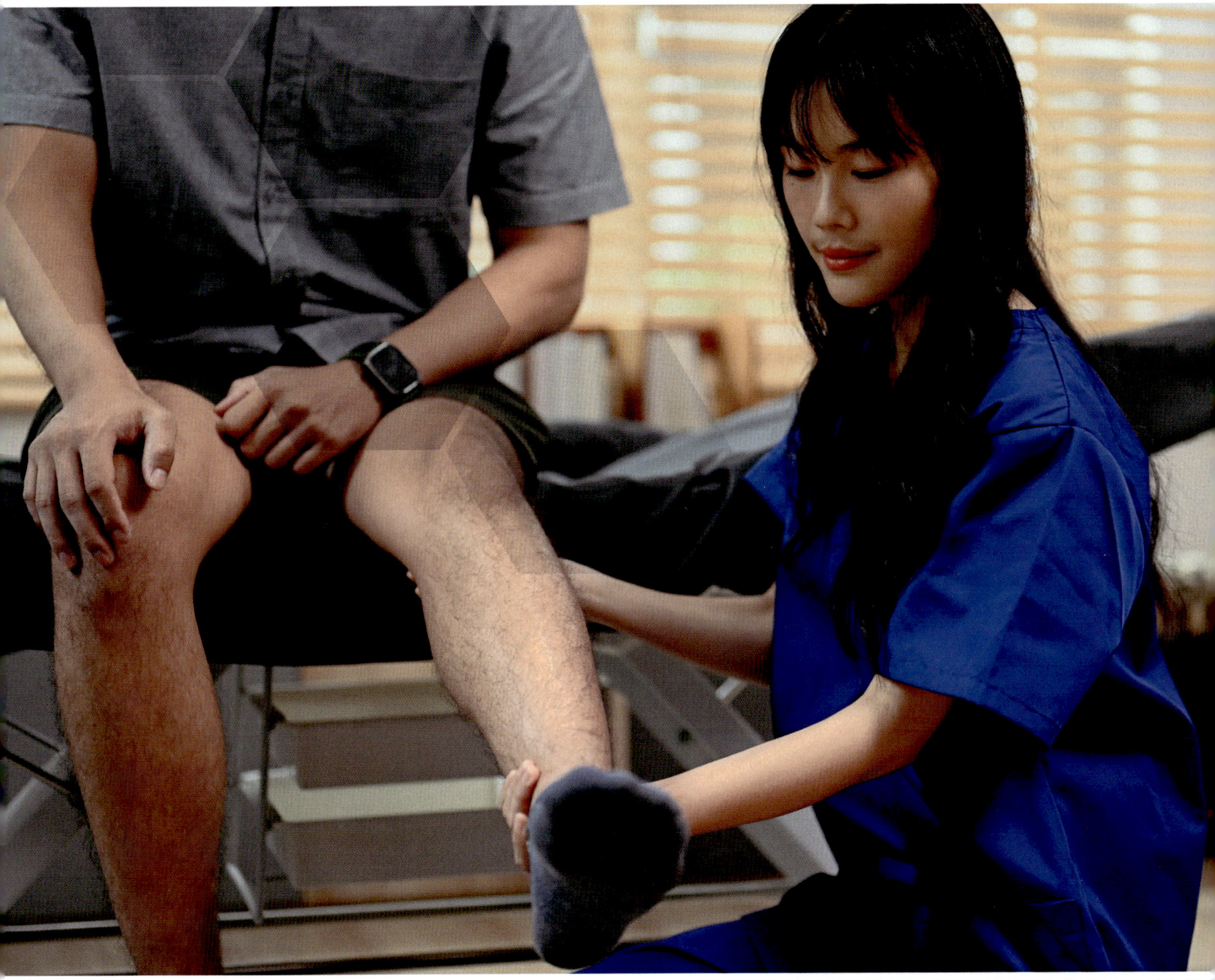

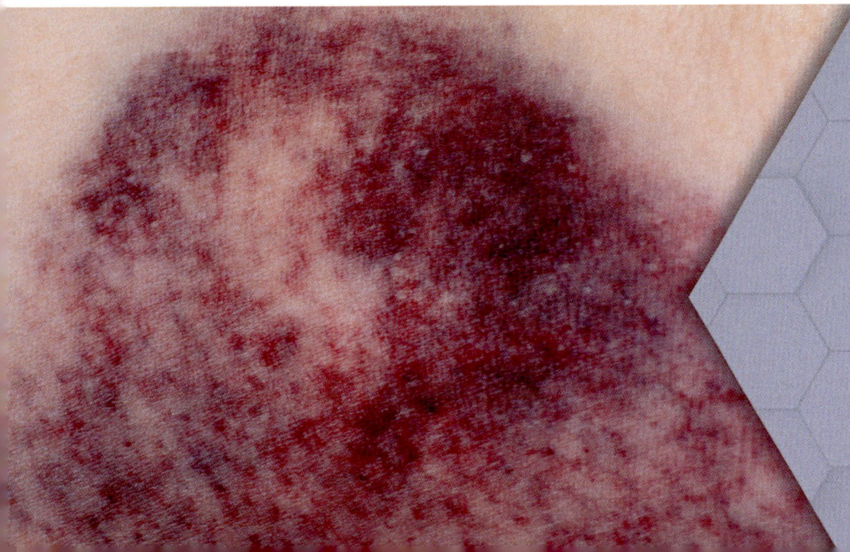

Medical professionals will also look at the injured leg. If the athlete is able to move the leg, the doctors or athletic trainer will examine the leg's range of motion. They will also see if there is any bruising or swelling. This will help them to determine what grade of injury an athlete has.

Additional Tests

Doctors may order additional tests to help them find out the severity of the injury.

Magnetic Resonance Imaging, commonly called MRI, is used to look at the muscle and soft tissue. An MRI uses radio waves produced by a computer and a strong magnetic field to create images of the inside of your body. This can help doctors find out the amount of tear in a muscle.

When MRIs were first invented, they were called NMR. That stands for Nuclear Magnetic Resonance. The name was changed, because many people were afraid of the word "nuclear".

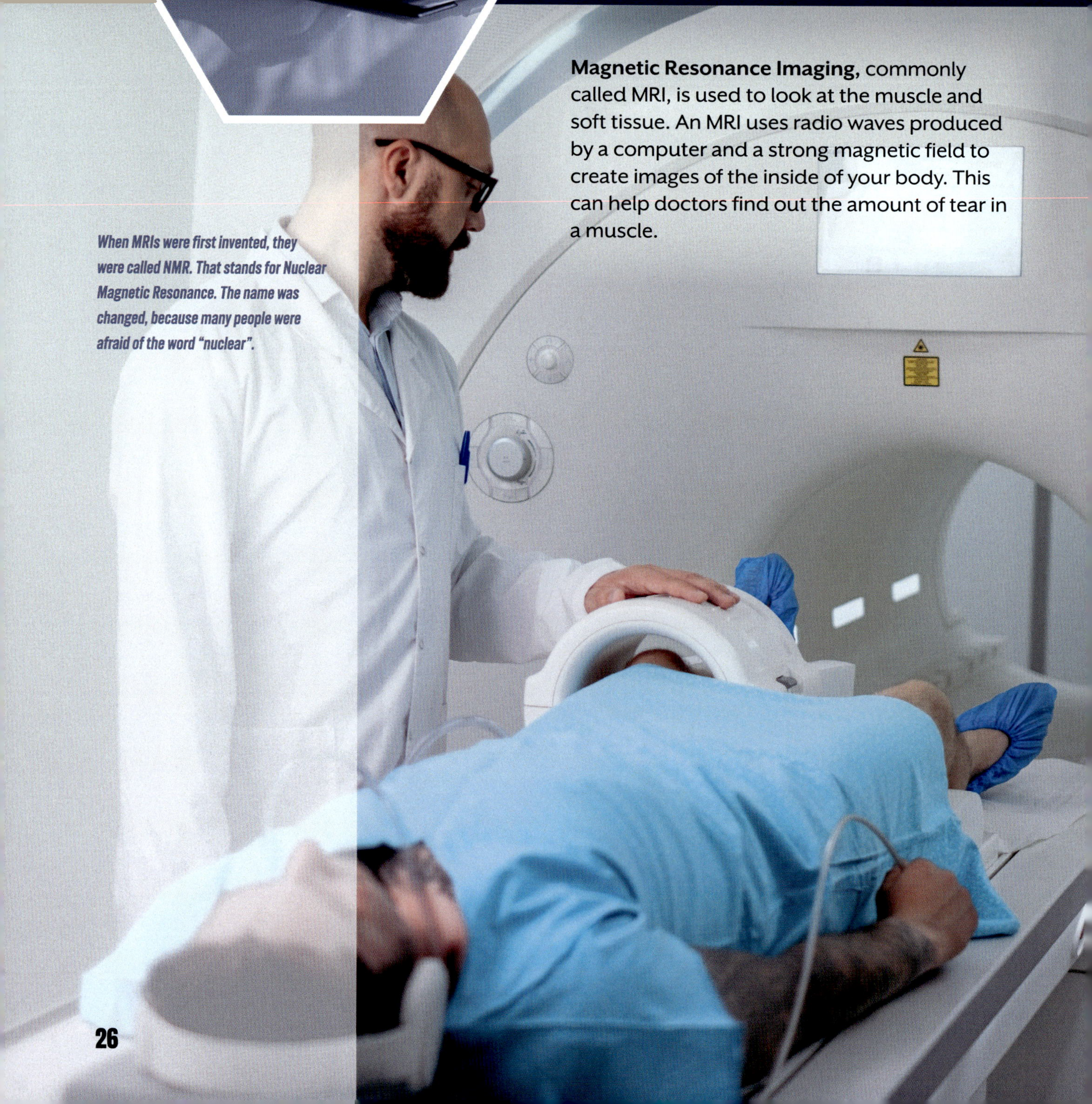

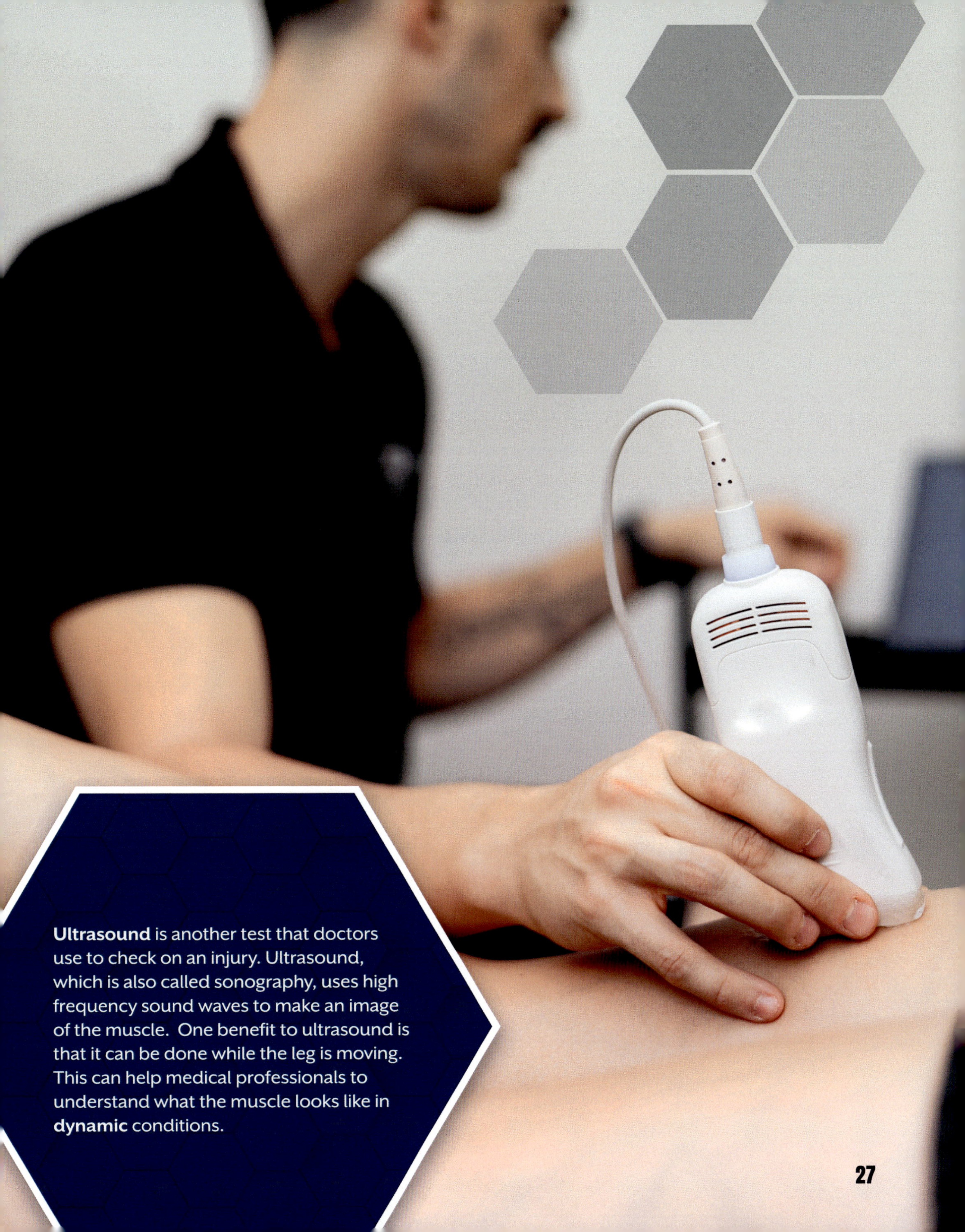

Ultrasound is another test that doctors use to check on an injury. Ultrasound, which is also called sonography, uses high frequency sound waves to make an image of the muscle. One benefit to ultrasound is that it can be done while the leg is moving. This can help medical professionals to understand what the muscle looks like in **dynamic** conditions.

Doctors may also use x-rays to examine the injury, especially if they suspect that there's a Grade 3 injury. X-rays take pictures of bone but don't show any muscle or other soft tissue such as tendons. Doctors use these images to see if parts of the bone have been removed during an avulsion injury.

Both MRIs and X-rays must be taken while the athlete is lying still.

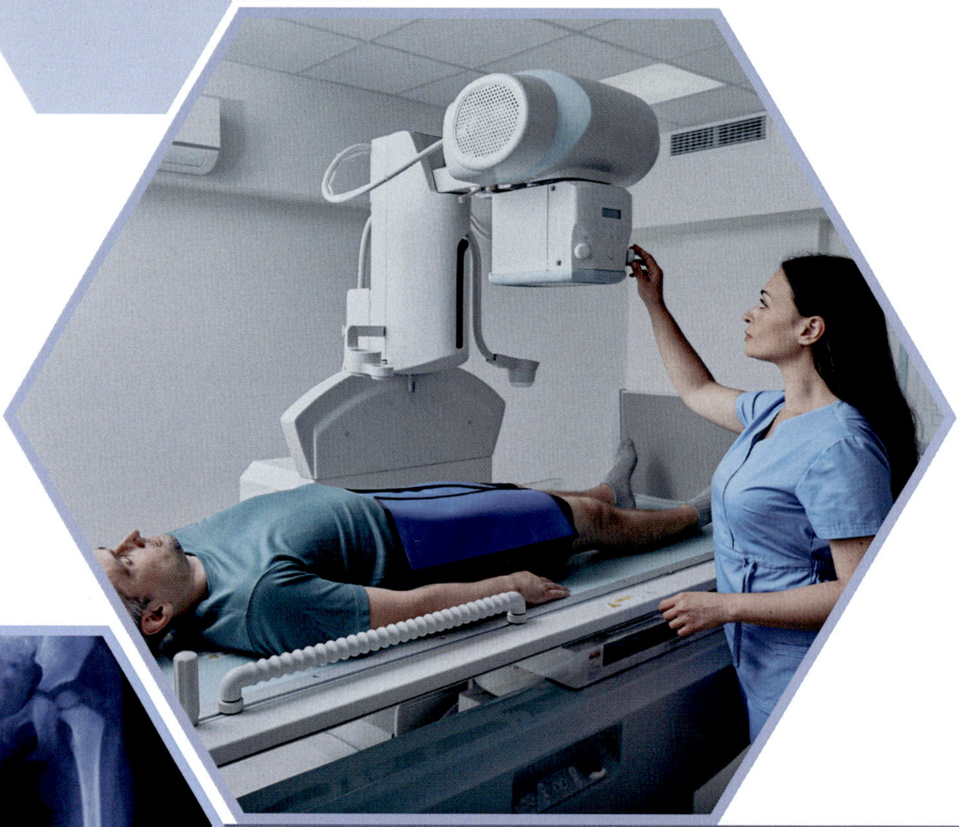

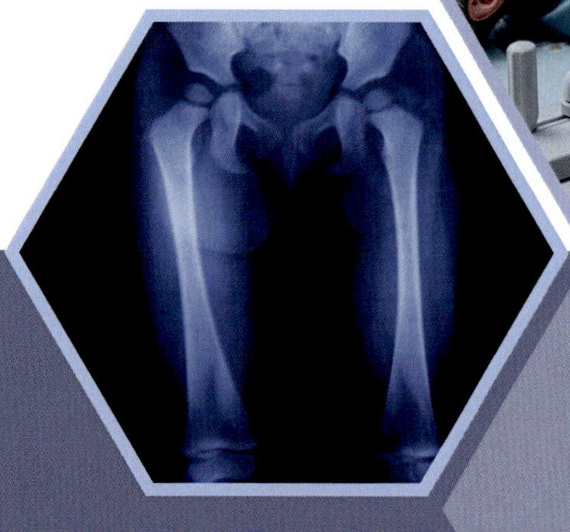

We know today that X-rays can be dangerous, but no one realized that when they were first discovered. Today, they're only used in places where there are a lot of safety precautions in place. However, it wasn't always this way. In the 1930s and 1940s, you could even have your foot X-rayed in a shoe store to see how your new shoe fit!

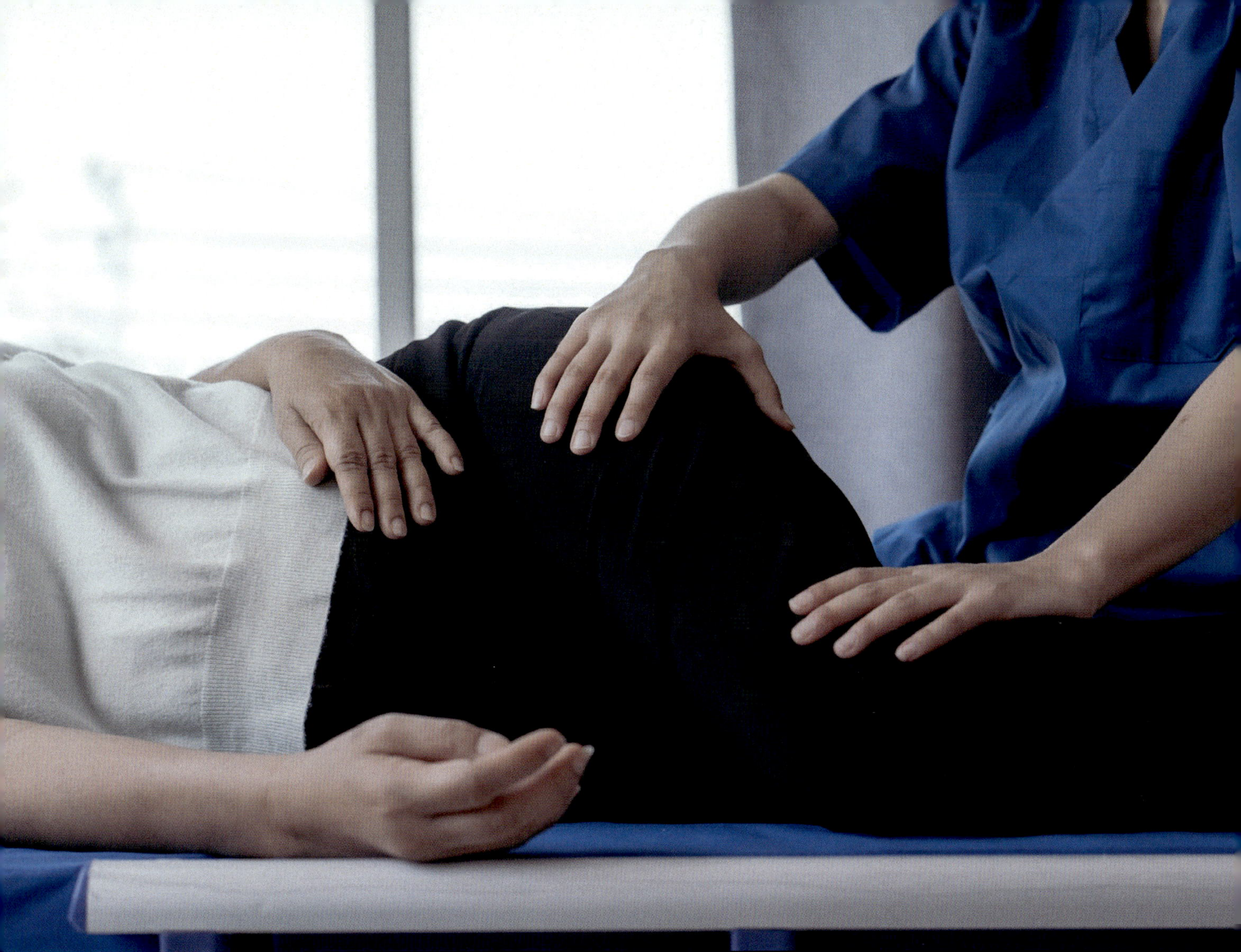

Chapter 6: Treatment

Hamstring injuries are treated in many ways. It's important for doctors or other medical professionals to determine how bad the athlete's injury is first. They will prescribe different methods of treatment based on the grade of injury.

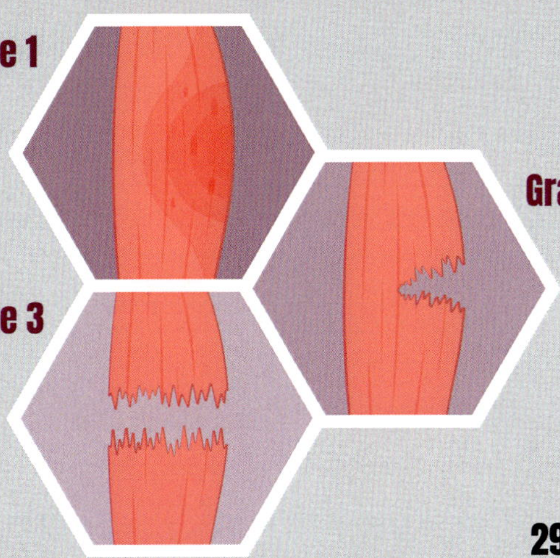

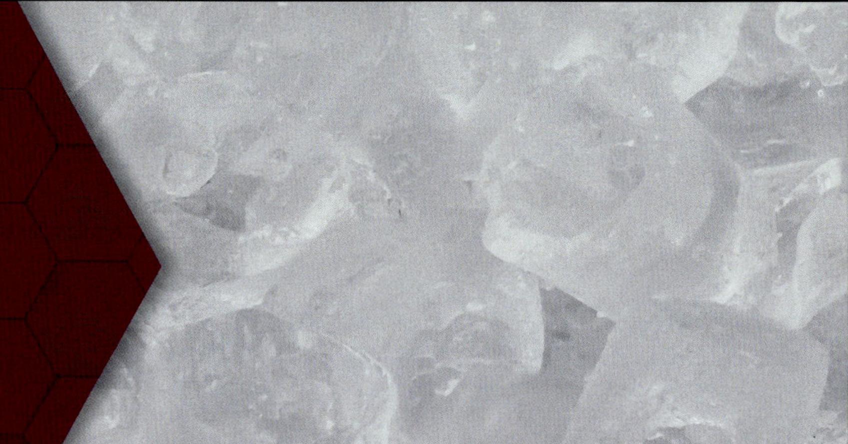

Most hamstring injuries will heal with simple treatment. Doctors and trainers may initially prescribe RICE to an injured athlete. RICE stands for

- Rest
- Ice
- Compression
- Elevation

RICE is one of the easiest and most effective ways to start treating muscle strain injuries.

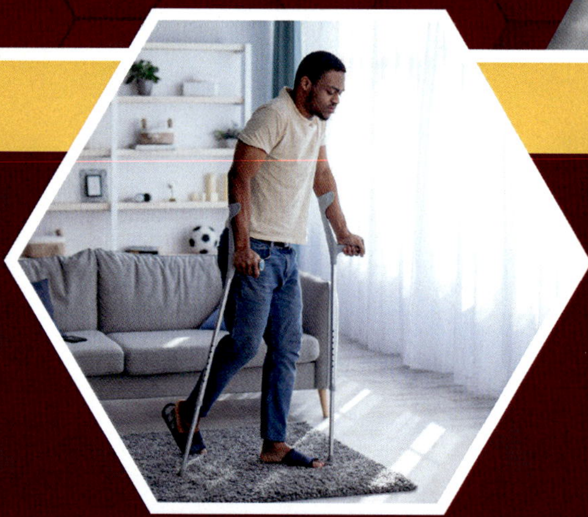

Rest

It is important to stop using the injured leg. The injured athlete should not try to play sports while hurt.

Ice

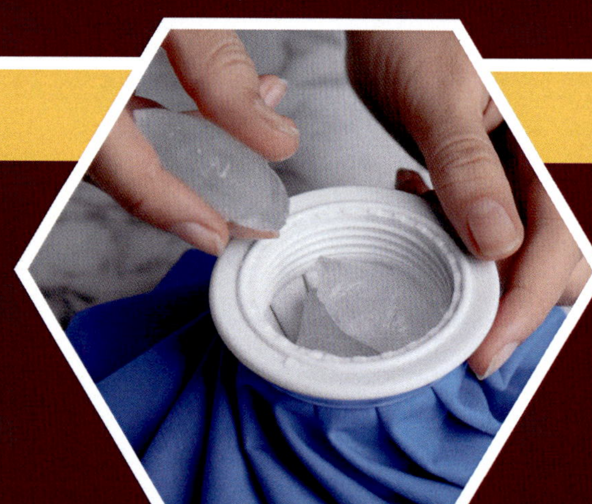

Ice helps to keep swelling down and to decrease pain in the injured area. Athletes should wrap ice packs in a cloth, rather than applying ice directly to their skin. After applying the ice for 20 minutes, the athlete should wait at least 20 minutes before applying ice again.

If your doctor tells you to ice an injury, they will also tell you how many times to apply the ice. Be sure to listen to your doctor's instructions so that you don't make the injury worse.

At some point during your recovery, your doctor or trainer may suggest that you use heat on your injury. Heat does the opposite of ice – it helps increase blood flow to your wound. It also can help your muscles and ligaments warm up and feel loose.

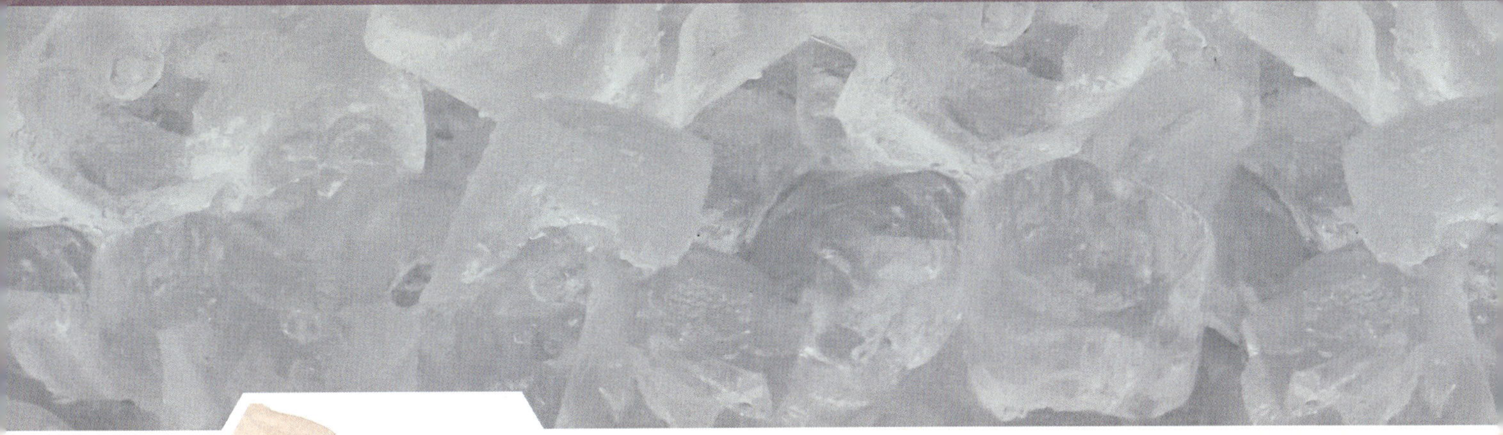

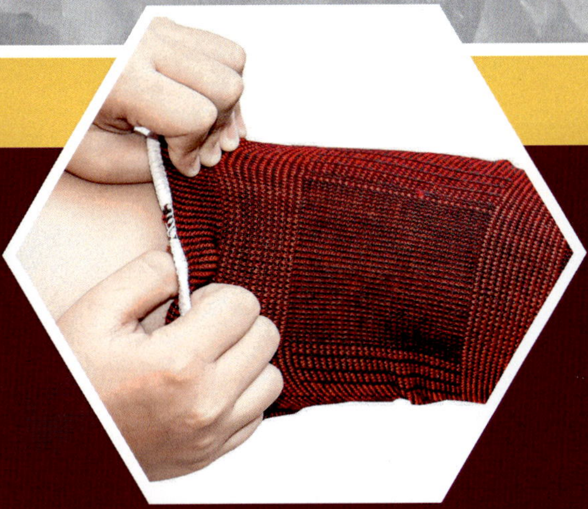

Compression

Compressing the injured muscle using an elastic bandage is another way to decrease swelling. If the injury includes an open wound, compression will also help to stop the loss of blood.

Elevation

Elevating the injured limb means raising it higher than the athlete's heart. For a hamstring injury, this means that the athlete should be lying down or sitting in order to raise the injured leg. Elevating the injury helps decrease swelling.

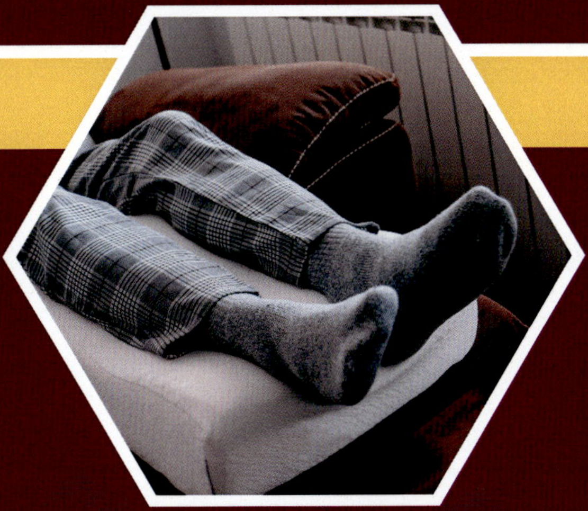

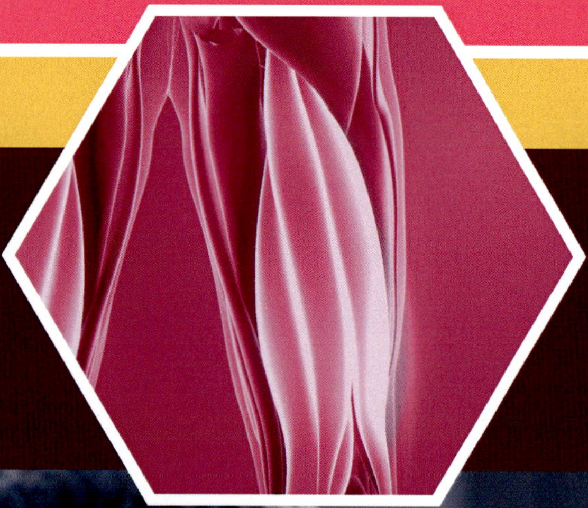

Surgery

Surgery is sometimes needed for hamstring injuries. Avulsion injuries are usually the only hamstring injuries that require surgery. During surgery for a hamstring injury, surgeons work to reattach the tendon to the bone using **bone anchors**.

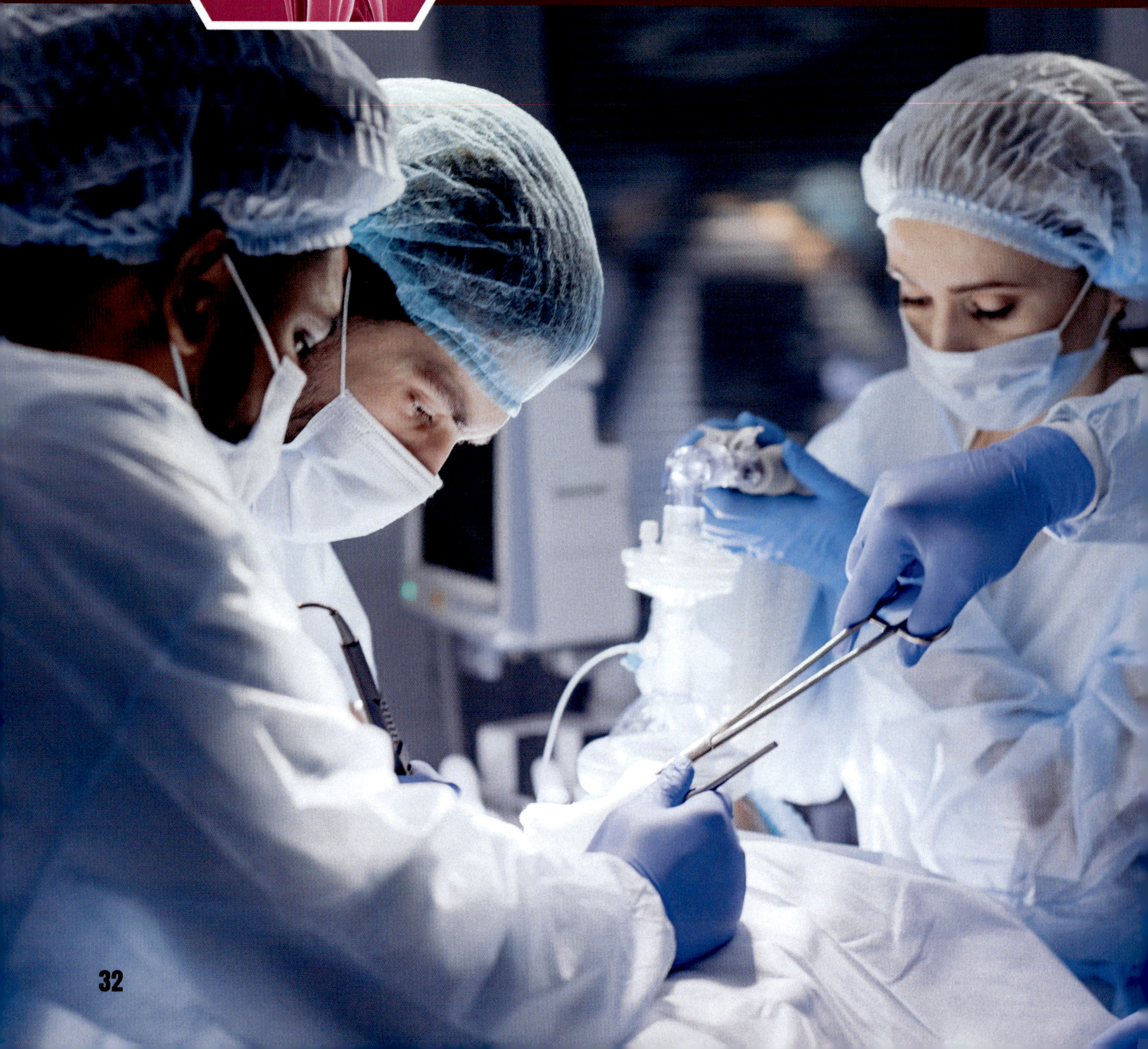

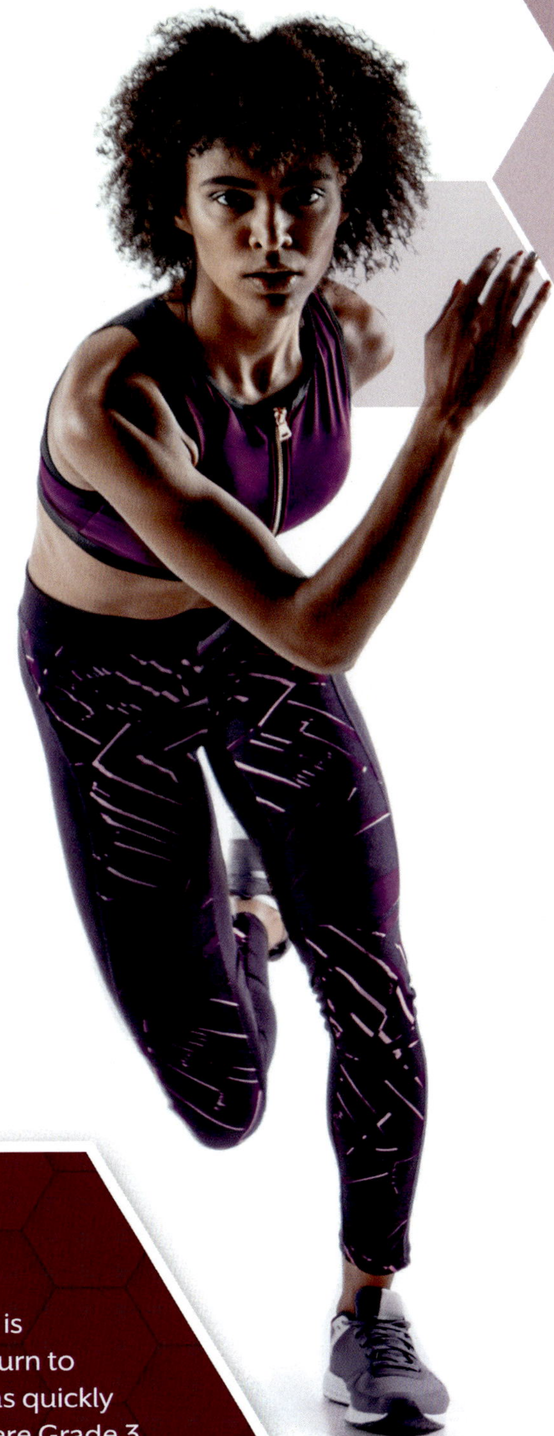

The goal of treatment is to help the athlete return to healthy playing form as quickly as possible. More severe Grade 3 injuries will take the longest time to heal, while less severe Grade 1 and 2 injuries will respond to treatment more quickly.

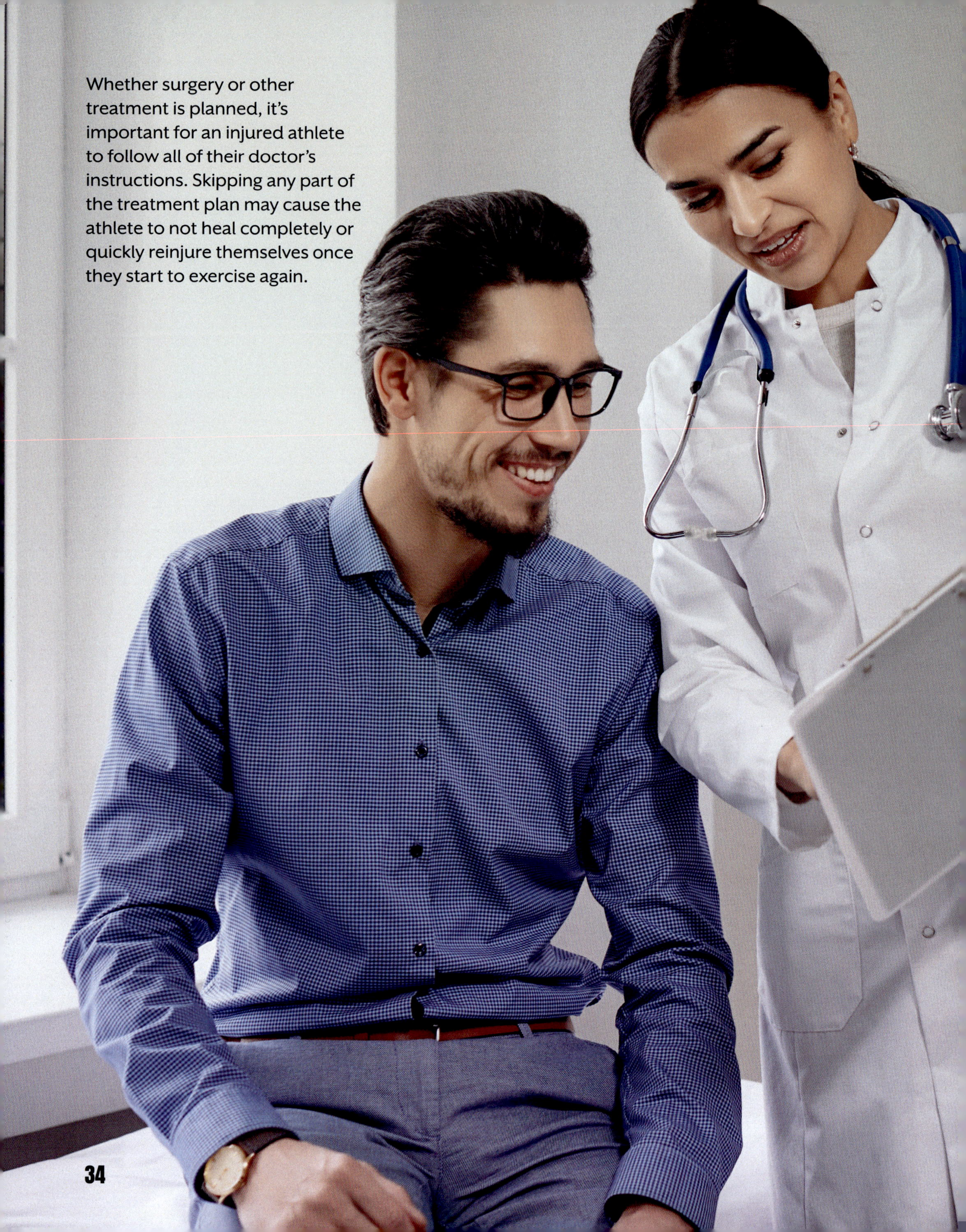

Whether surgery or other treatment is planned, it's important for an injured athlete to follow all of their doctor's instructions. Skipping any part of the treatment plan may cause the athlete to not heal completely or quickly reinjure themselves once they start to exercise again.

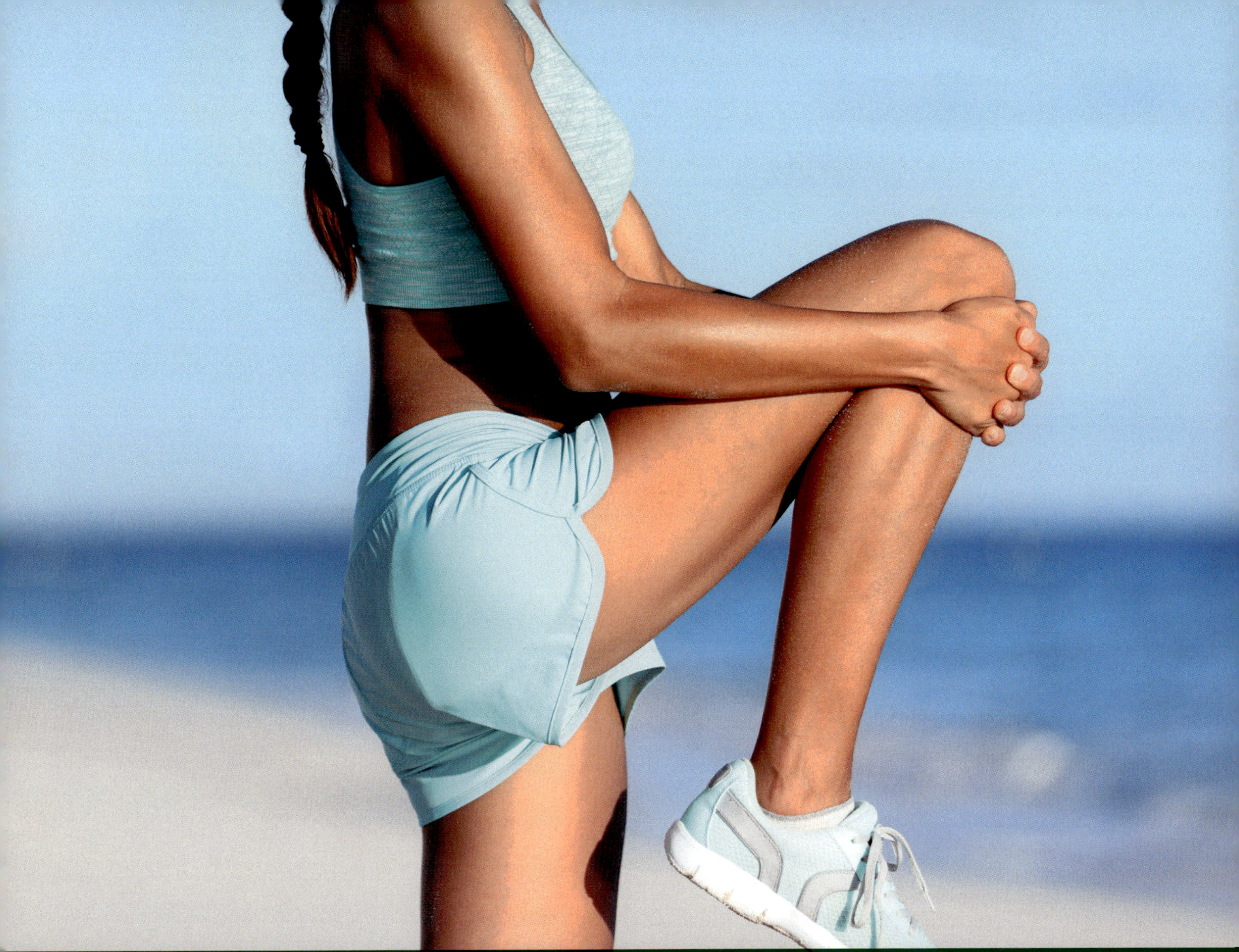

Chapter 7: Recovery

Many hamstring injuries will heal on their own. However, it may take a long time for the injury to heal completely. Low grade injuries may heal in several days while more severe, Grade 2 or 3 injuries may take weeks or months to heal completely.

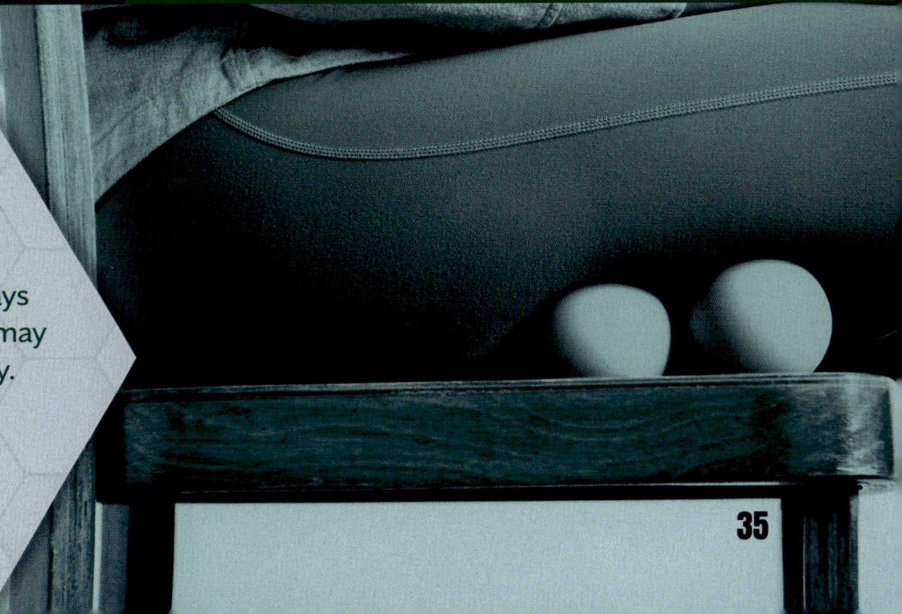

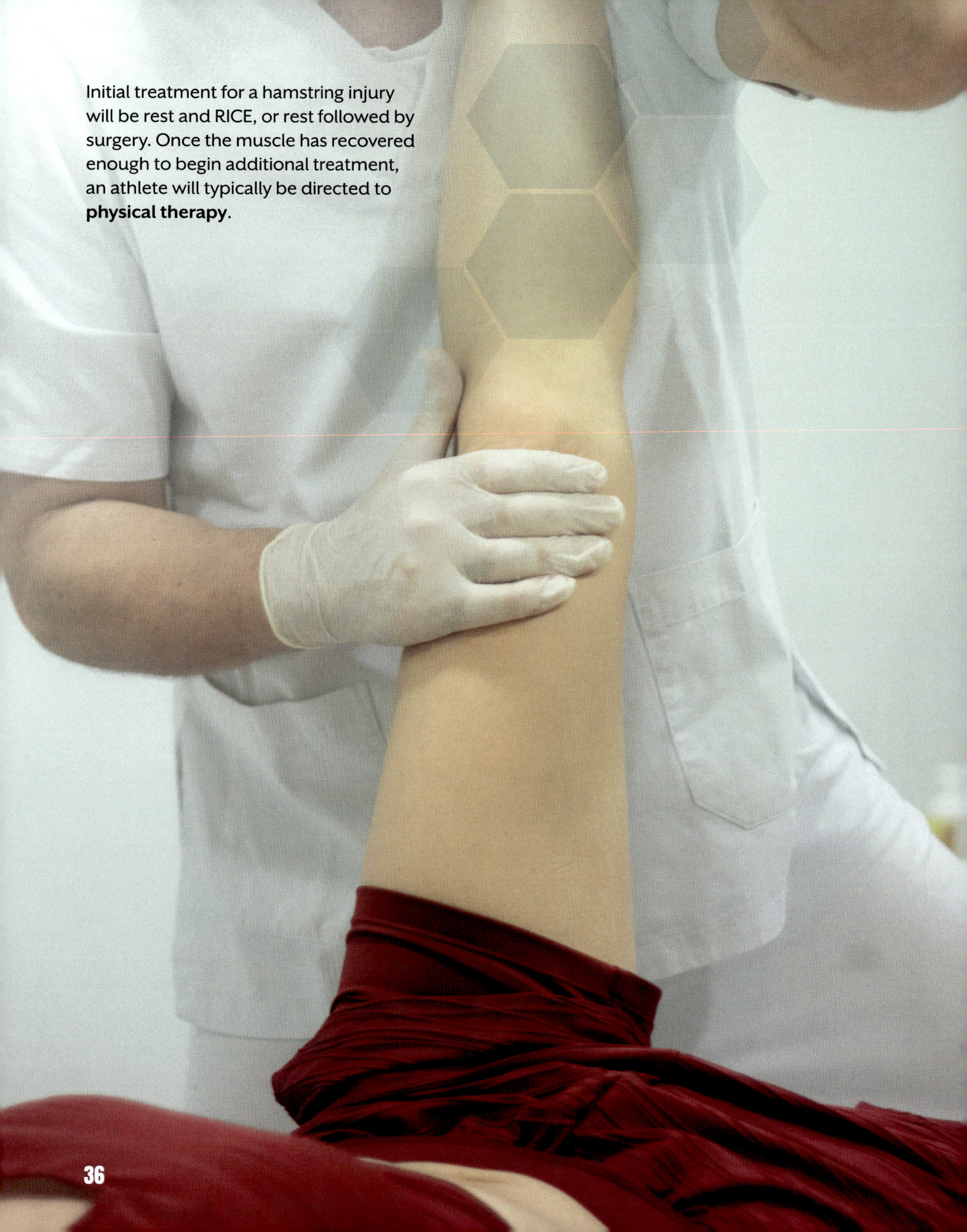

Initial treatment for a hamstring injury will be rest and RICE, or rest followed by surgery. Once the muscle has recovered enough to begin additional treatment, an athlete will typically be directed to **physical therapy**.

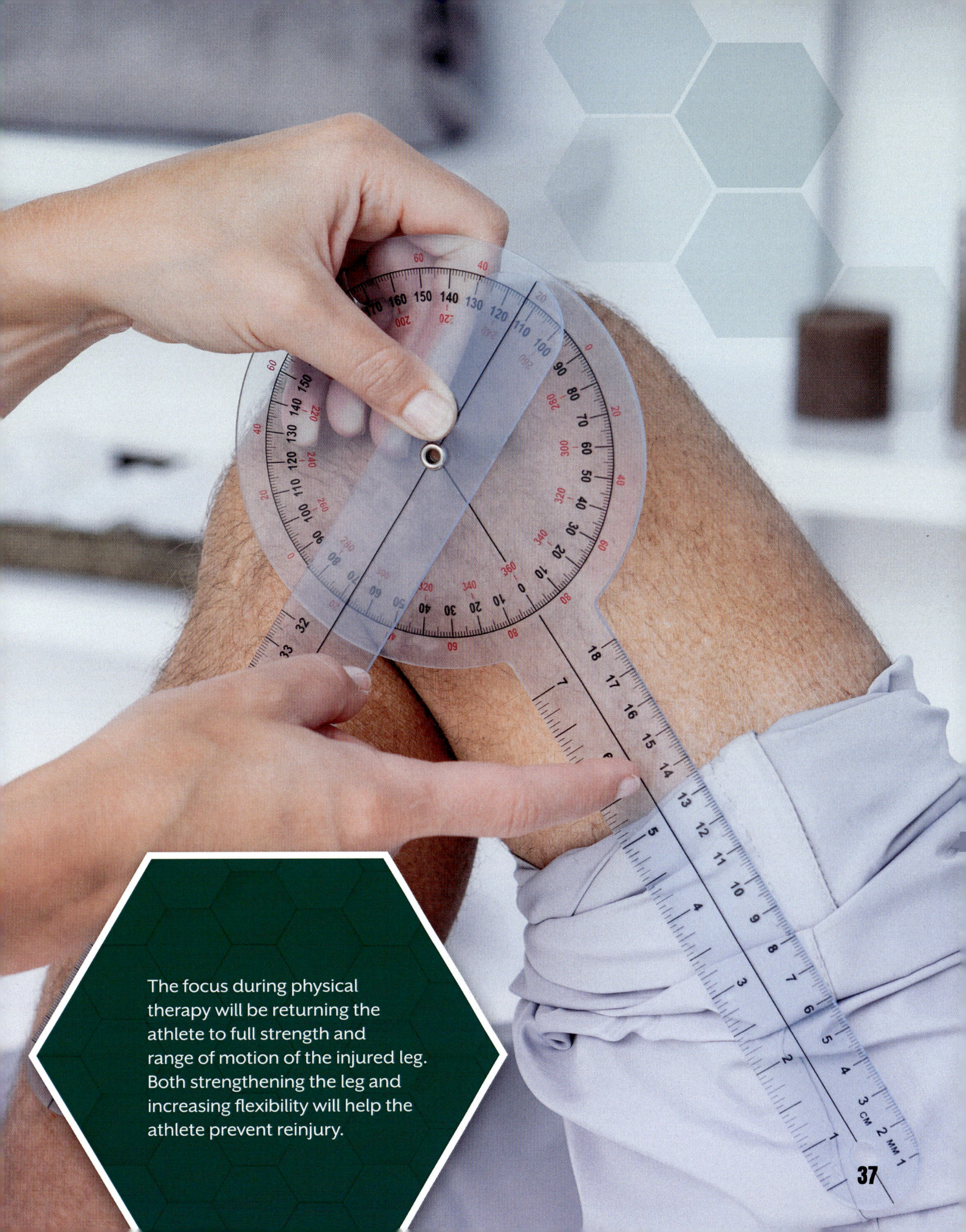

The focus during physical therapy will be returning the athlete to full strength and range of motion of the injured leg. Both strengthening the leg and increasing flexibility will help the athlete prevent reinjury.

Stretches

Physical therapists will help the injured athlete develop a stretching routine. Some stretches will be **static**, meaning that the athlete will sit, stand, or lay down in one position during the stretch. Other stretches will be **dynamic**, meaning that the athlete will stretch during controlled movement.

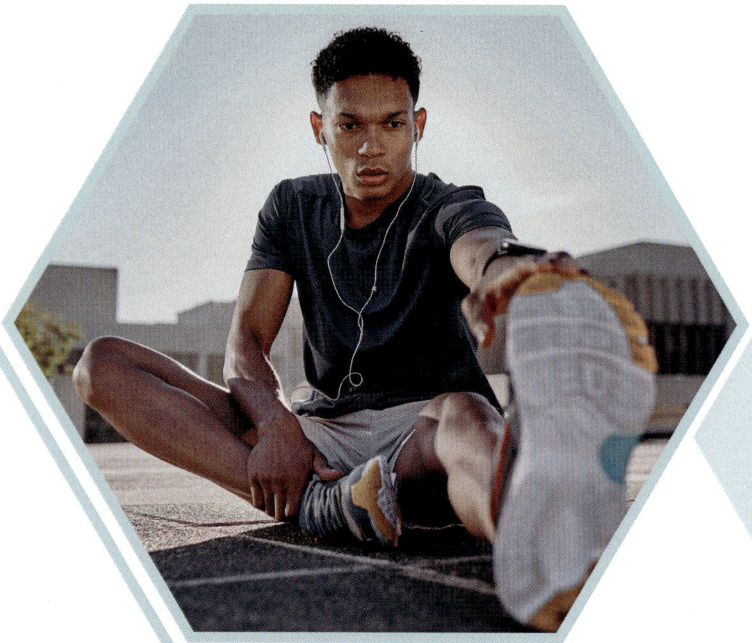

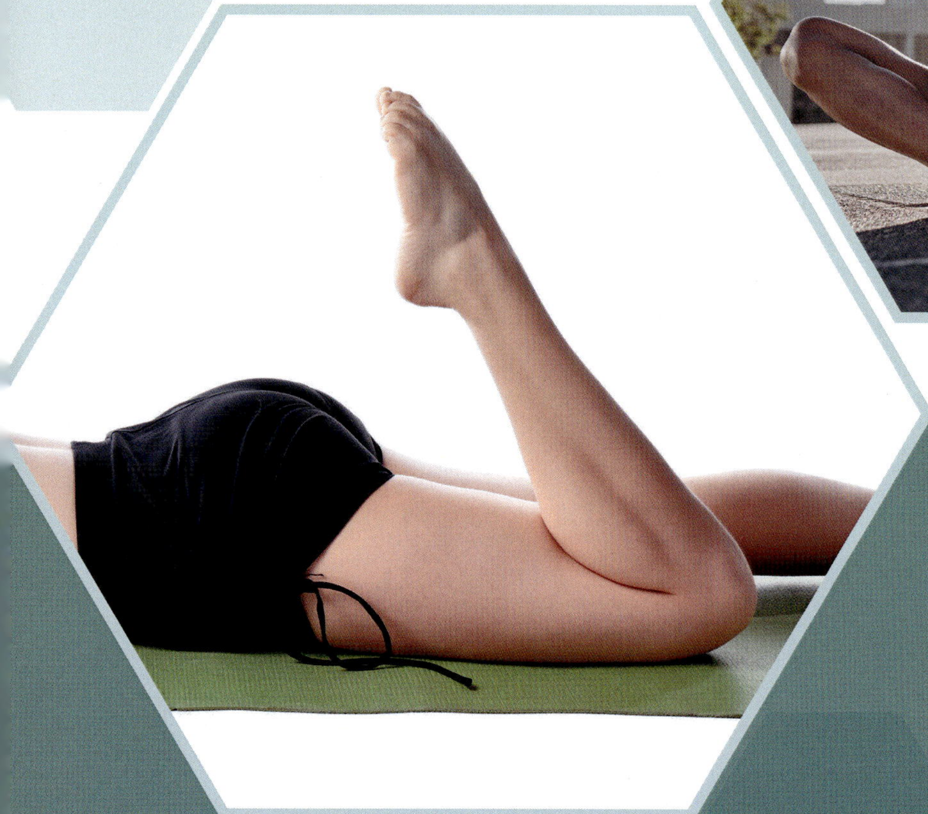

One exercise a physical therapist may suggest is a prone hamstring curl.

1.) *Lay on your stomach with your feet hanging off of a bed*
2.) *Slowly bend your knee to 90 degrees*
3.) *Slowly lower your leg down*

Strength training

Strengthening the hamstring and leg muscles will be part of an athlete's recovery from a hamstring injury. However, it is important for the athlete to strengthen other parts of their body as well. Working to increase the strength of core muscles will help an athlete control their movements and decrease the strain on the hamstring muscles.

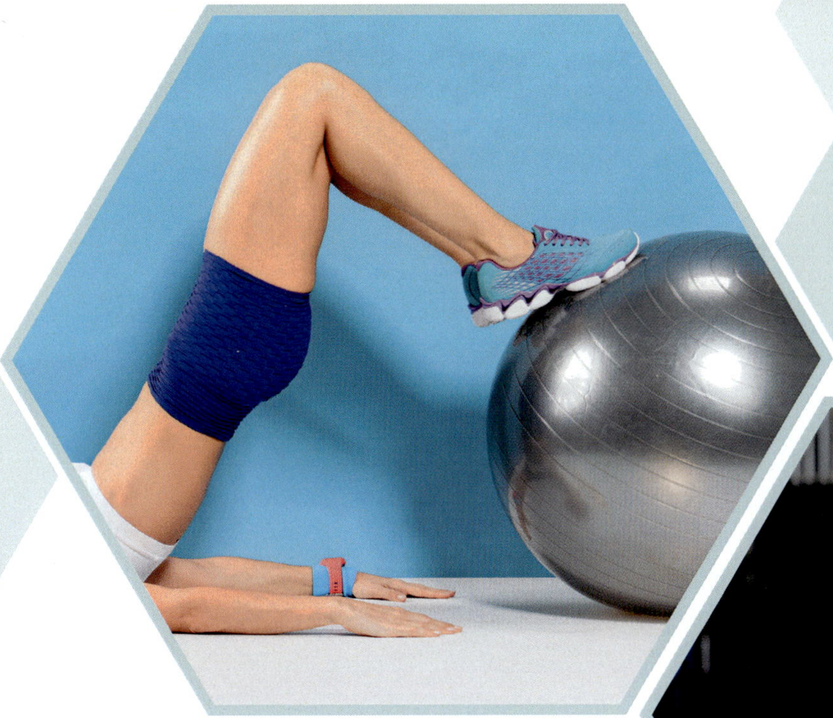

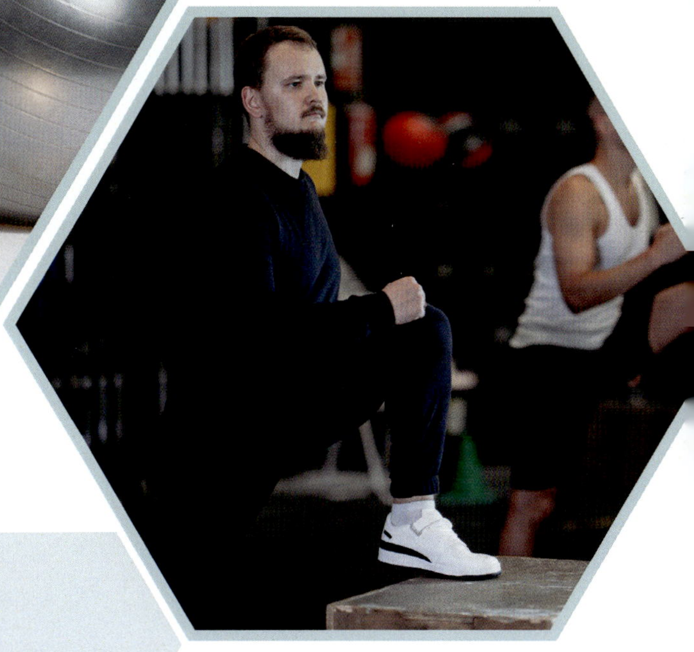

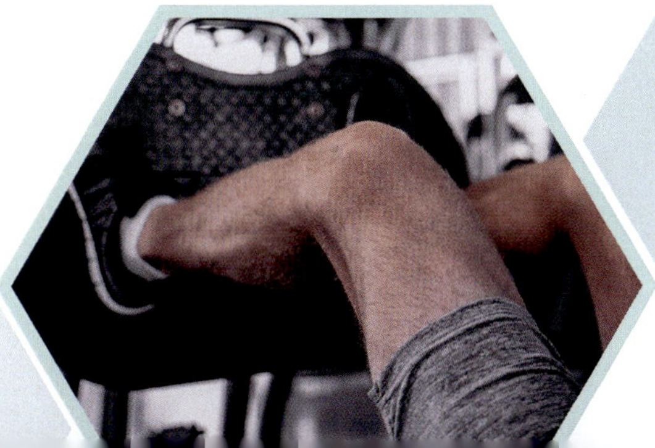

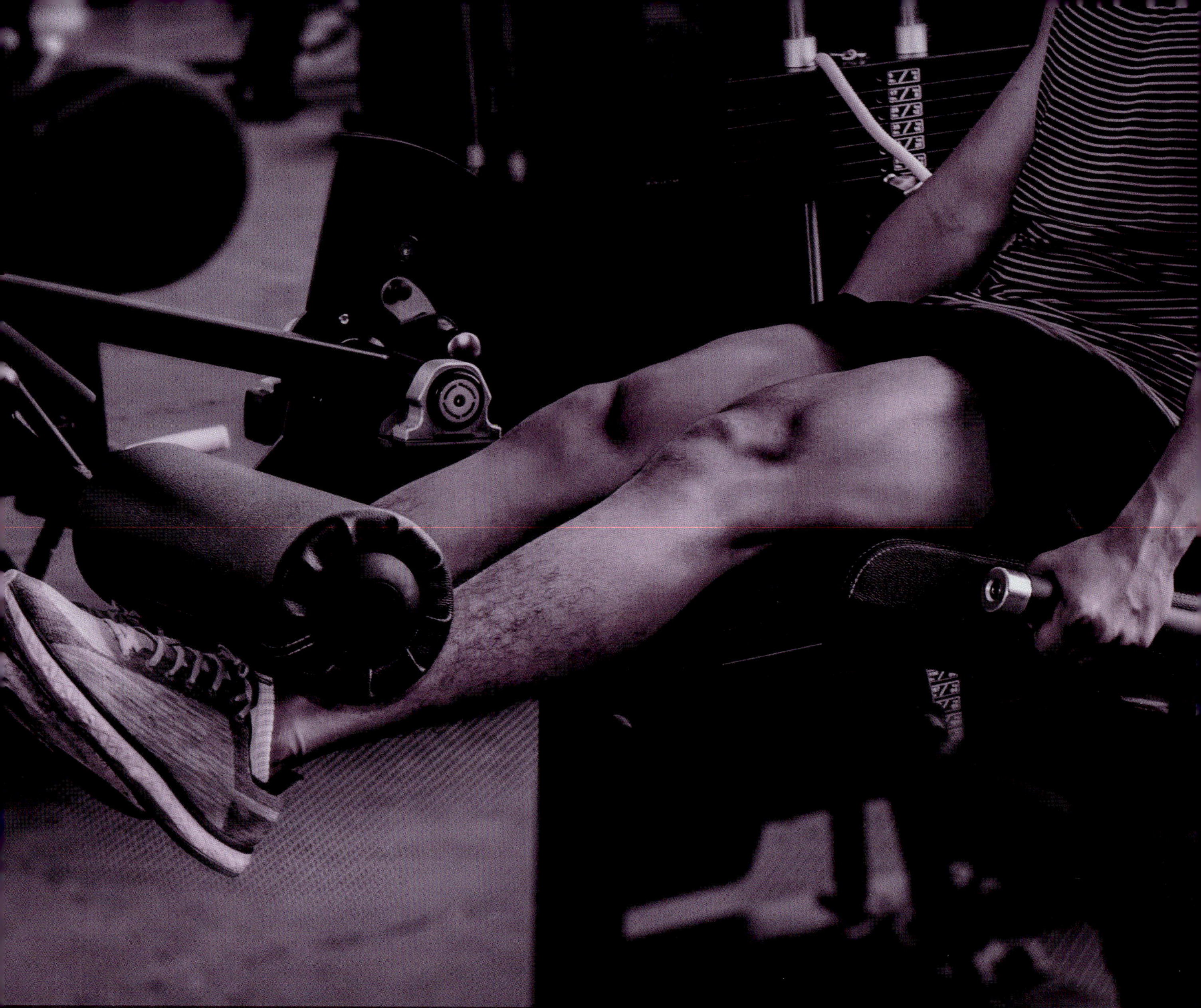

Chapter 8: Prevention

Many athletes are likely to reinjure their hamstrings. One-third of athlete who have a hamstring injury will reinjure themselves within a year. Working to prevent hamstring injuries is an important part of being a healthy athlete.

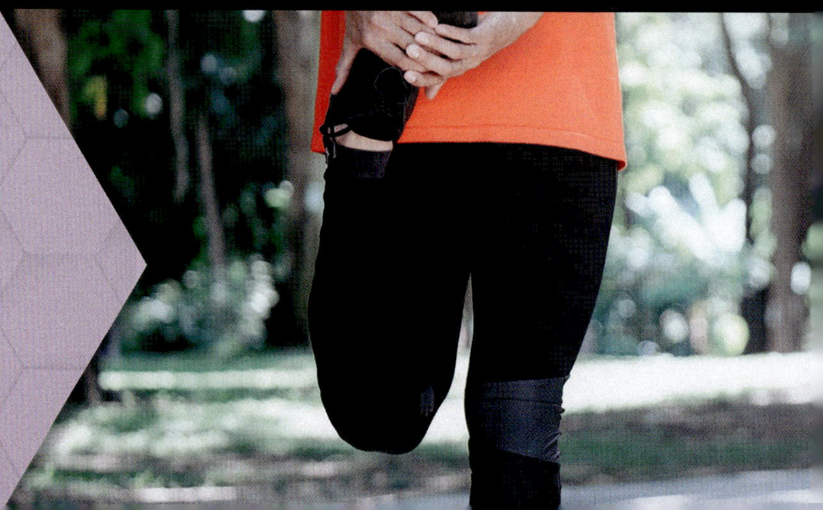

One of the leading causes of hamstring injury is when muscles don't have a lot of flexibility. A stiff muscle tears more easily than a loose, flexible muscle. Athletes should include stretches in their normal workout routines.

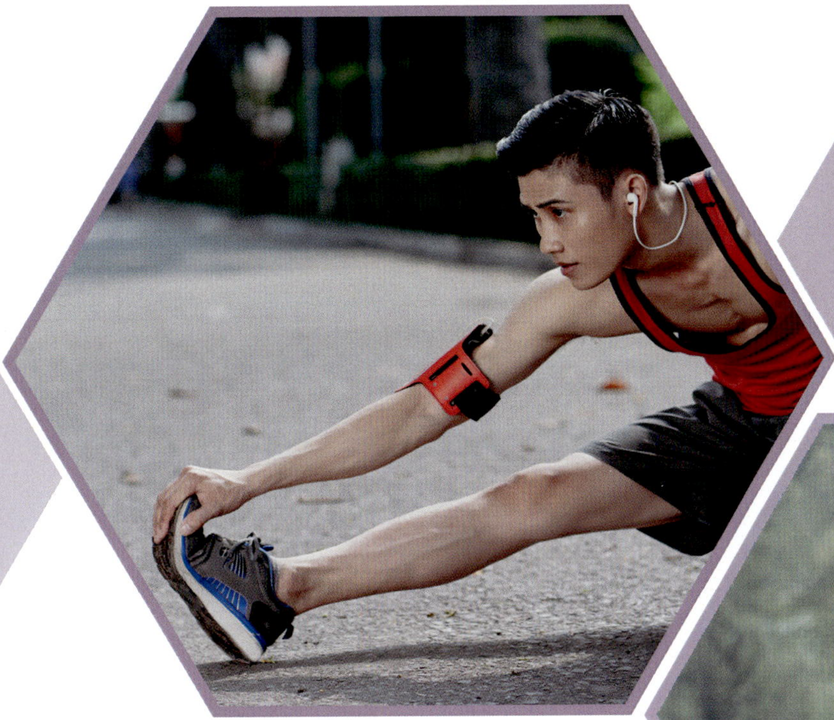

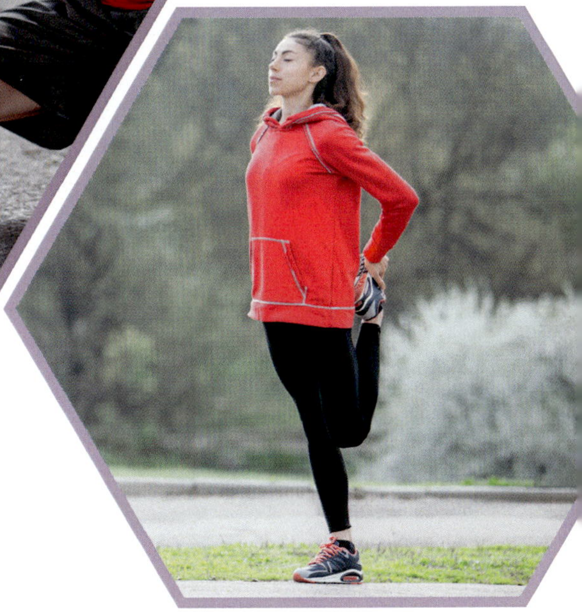

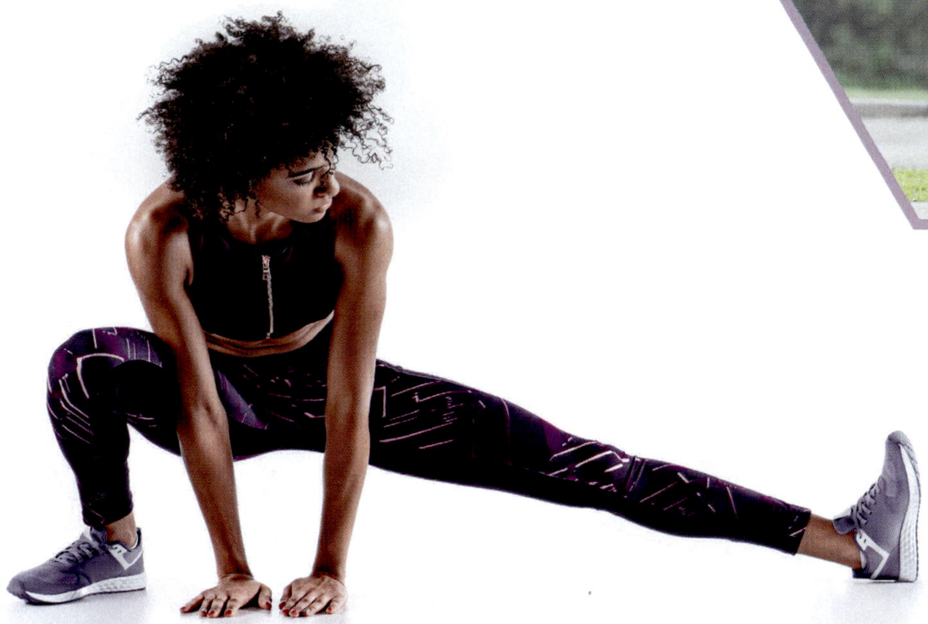

Another way to help the hamstring muscles stay flexible is to follow a good warm-up routine. One great way to warm up the hamstrings is with the "butt kick" exercise. While slowly jogging, try kicking your heel all the way back to your butt. Your hamstrings are some of the main muscles activating during this exercise. Taking time to warm up helps the muscles to loosen before strenuous exercise.

It is also important to take the time to cool down and stretch after exercising as well. This will increase the flexibility of the hamstring muscles and make them less likely to tear the next time you exercise.

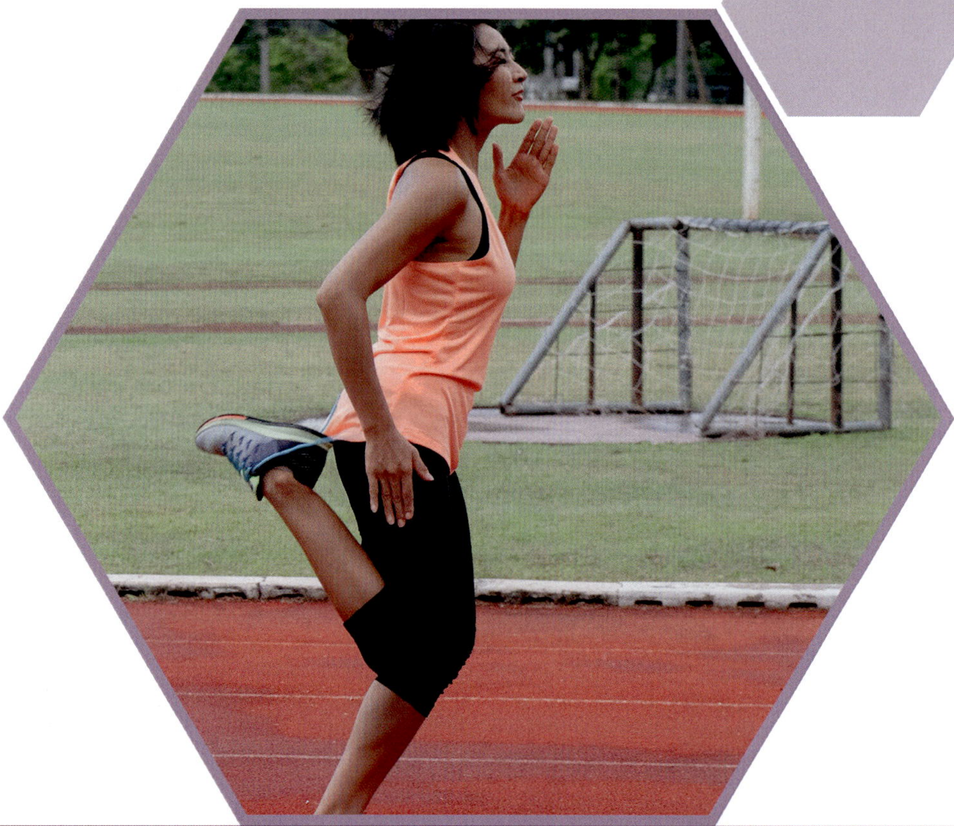

If you have pain in your lower back, a doctor or physical therapist may suggest exercises to strengthen your hamstrings. The hamstring muscles connect to your pelvis and can tilt your pelvis. Making these muscles strong can help your back be strong, too!

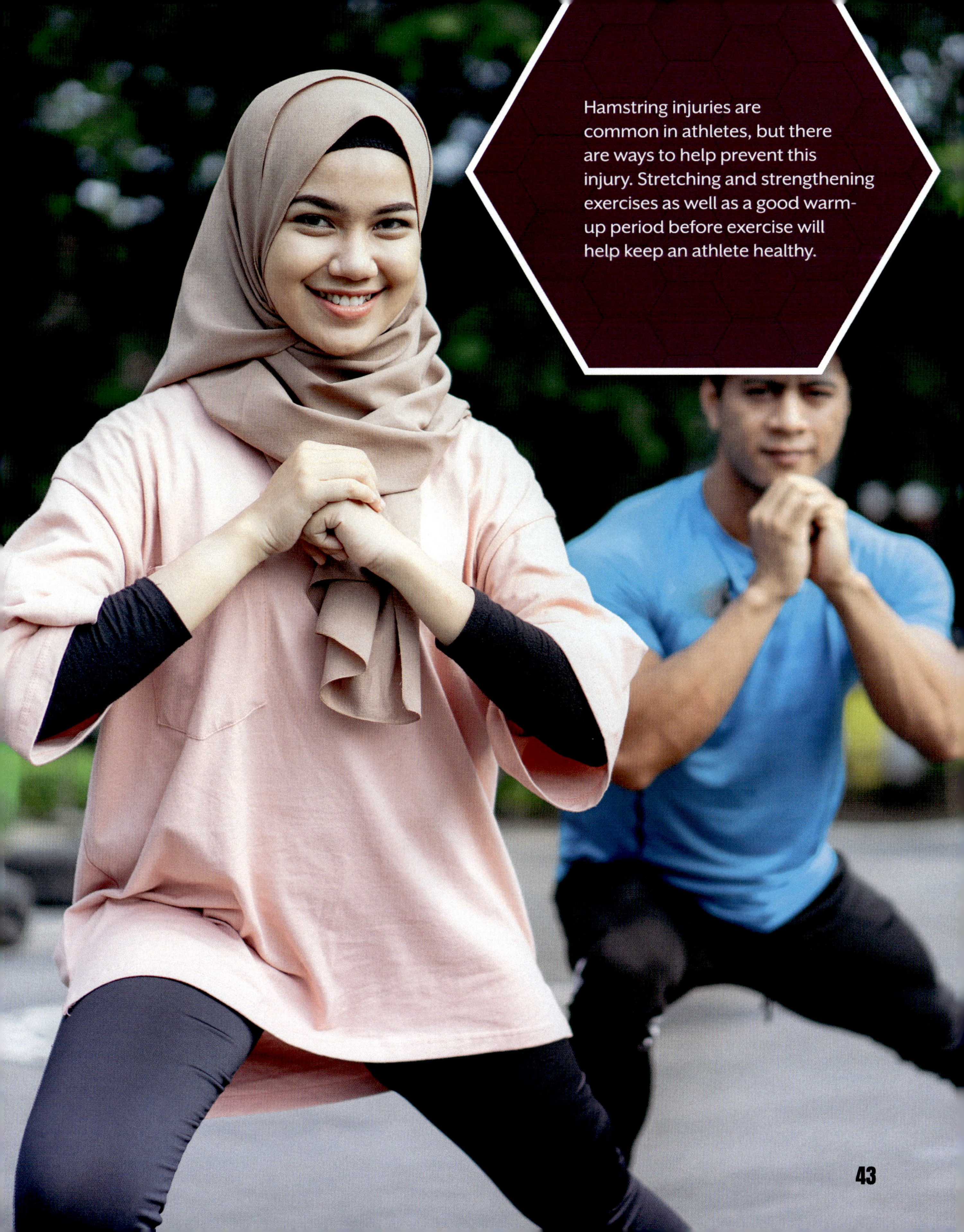

Hamstring injuries are common in athletes, but there are ways to help prevent this injury. Stretching and strengthening exercises as well as a good warm-up period before exercise will help keep an athlete healthy.

Glossary

acute injury (uh-KYOOT IN-juh-ree): An injury that happens suddenly

anatomy (un-NAT-uh-mee): The study of the parts of the human body

avulsion injury (uh-VUHL-shun IN-juh-ree): An injury where part of the bone is torn away

biceps femoris (BHAY-seps FEM-er-is): One of the three hamstrings muscles. This muscle a long head and a short head and attaches to the fibula

bone (bohn): A hard material in the human body that provides structure

bone anchor (bohn ANG-ker): A tool used during surgery to attach tendon to bone

dynamic (dhay-NAM-ik): In motion

eccentric contraction (ik-SEN-trik kuhn-TRAK-shun): When muscles exert energy while lengthening

femur (FEE-mur): The upper leg bone and the longest bone in the human body

joint (joint): Where two or more bones meet

ligaments (LIG-uh-muhnts): Soft structures which connect bones with other bones

magnetic resonance imaging (mag-NET-ik REZ-uh-nuhns IM-uh-jing): A machine that uses magnets to take images of the soft parts inside the human body, commonly known as MRI

mobile joint (MOH-buhl joint): A joint whose purpose is to move

muscles (MUH-sels): Soft tissue in the human body which contracts to move bones

pelvis (PEL-vis): A group of bones that make up the lower torso, commonly known as the hip bones

physical therapy (FIZ-i-kuhl THER-uh-pee): A branch of medicine that helps patients regain and main health through exercises and stretches

range of motion (reynj uhv MOH-shun): How far a joint is able to move

semimembranosus (SEM-i-MEM-brah-noh-sus): One of the three hamstrings muscles. This muscle begins on the pelvis and ends on the tibia and knee ligaments

semitendinosus (SEM-i-TEN-duhn-noh-sus): One of the three hamstrings muscles. This muscle beings on the pelvis and ends on the tibia

static (stat-ik): Without motion

tendon (TEN-duhn): The soft structure that connects muscle and bone

tibia (TIB-ee-uh): The long bone of the lower leg. This is commonly called the shin bone

ultrasound (UHL-truh-sound): High frequency sound waves that are used to see inside the human body

Index

Comprehension Questions

1. How many muscles are in the hamstring complex?
   a. 1
   b. 3
   c. 5
2. True or false: Hamstring injuries are common sports injuries.
3. The two heads of the biceps femoris muscle are
   a. long and short.
   b. big and little.
   c. thick and thin.
4. True or false: Nerve damage is necessary to have an avulsion injury
5. True or false: Grade 3 hamstring injuries are the most severe.
6. RICE stands for
   a. Running, Ice skating, Climbing, and Equestrian.
   b. Red, Inflamed, Contusion, and Enlarged.
   c. Rest, Ice, Compression, and Elevation.
7. One way to prevent hamstring injuries is to
   a. drink milk.
   b. stretch before exercising.
   c. only exercise on artificial turf.
8. True or false: Athletes who have one hamstring injury are likely to have another.

1. b 2. true 3. a 4. false 5. true 6. c 7. b 8. true

About the Author

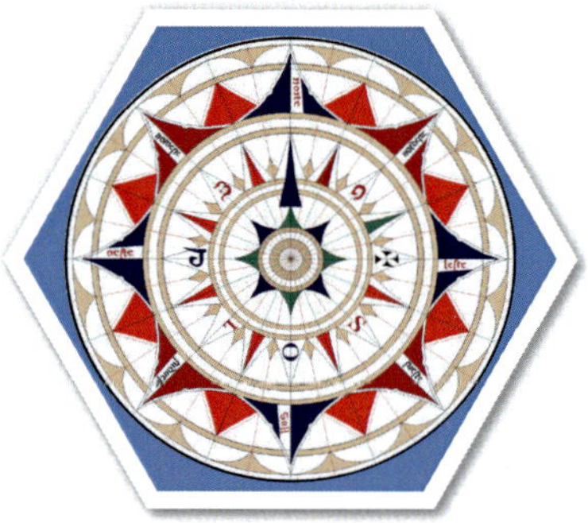

India James writes about science, technology, and math for young readers. She loves when science comes together with sports. India lives in Ohio with her family.

Author: India James

Editor: Ellen Rodger

Design: Jen Bowers

IMAGE CREDITS

Shutterstock: Cover and title page ©2024 Cinefootage Visuals (p.4, p.11, p.32), ©2012 Maxisport (p.12), ©2022 Studio Romantic (p.5), ©2019 AYA images (p.7); p.4 ©2023 Hananeko_Studio; p.5 ©2018 PhotoProCorp; p.6 ©2018 Alizada Studios, ©2017 Andre Gie; p.7 ©2018 OSTILL is Franck Camhi; p.8 ©2019 Orla; p.9 ©2014 Dirima, ©VectorMine; p.10 ©2022 PeopleImages.com-Yuri A, ©2016 Maridav; p.11 ©2021 PanicAttack; p.13 ©2014 Chad Zuber, ©2019 Regreto; p.14 ©medicalstocks; p.15 ©VectorPlotnikoff, ©2019 TndmAgency_Yuliia Zatula, ©2022 A.RICARDO; p.16 ©2018 Jacob Lund; p.17 ©2019 Mr.Louis (p.23), ©2022 Media Lens King; p.18 ©Pepermpron, ©2022 PeopleImages.com-Yuri A; p.19 ©Pepermpron, ©2014 Chad Zuber; p.20 ©Pepermpron, ©2021 Andrey_Popov; p.21 ©medicalstocks; p.22 ©2019 Andrey_Popov, ©2021 DC Studio; p.23 ©2021 Boonlert Saikrajang; p.24 ©2023 Dragon Images; p.25 ©2024 Prathankarnpap, ©2019 Lumena; p.26 ©2021 fizkes, ©2019 Nejron Photo; p.27 ©2023 Yiistocking; p.28 ©2022 Peakstock, ©2014 Puwadol Jaturawutthichai; p.29 ©2023 PanuShot, ©Pepermpron; p.30 ©2020 Wira SHK, ©2021 Prostock-studio, ©2019 New Africa; p.31 ©2014 Tewan Banditrakkanka, ©2023 nito; p.32 ©2018 UfaBizPhoto; p.33 ©2017 RomarioIen; p.34 ©2023 Studio Romantic; p.35 ©2021 Maridav, ©2023 pixie_mfr; p.36 ©2019 edwardolive; p.37 ©2015 wavebreakmedia; p.38 ©2022 PeopleImages com-Yuri A, ©2020 Fab_1; p.39 ©2020 Marcelo Trad, ©2024 BearFotos, ©2020 Maridav; p.40 ©2018 Love Solutions, ©2021 iJeab; p.41 ©2016 Dragon Images, ©2016 fizkes, ©2017 RomarioIen; p.42 ©2017 psgxxx; p.43 ©2021 Odua Images; p.48 About the Author image ©Alvesgaspar

Crabtree Publishing

crabtreebooks.com 800-387-7650

In Canada: We acknowledge the financial support of the Government of Canada through the Canada Book Fund for our publishing activities.

Hardcover 978-1-0398-8078-8
Paperback 978-1-0398-8439-7
Ebook (pdf) 978-1-0398-8198-3
Epub 978-1-0398-8318-5

Published in Canada
Crabtree Publishing
616 Welland Avenue
St. Catharines, Ontario
L2M 5V6

Published in the United States
Crabtree Publishing
347 Fifth Avenue
Suite 1402-145
New York, New York, 10016

Library and Archives Canada Cataloguing in Publication
Available at Library and Archives Canada

Library of Congress Cataloging-in-Publication Data
Available at the Library of Congress

Printed in the USA/CP2025